Narcisse Doune

Prognosis of heart failure in sub-Saharan Africa

Narcisse Doune

Prognosis of heart failure in sub-Saharan Africa

ScienciaScripts

Cover image: www.ingimage.com

This book is a translation from the original published under ISBN 978-620-6-72089-8.

Publisher:
Sciencia Scripts
is a trademark of
Dodo Books Indian Ocean Ltd. and OmniScriptum S.R.L publishing group

120 High Road, East Finchley, London, N2 9ED, United Kingdom
Str. Armeneasca 28/1, office 1, Chisinau MD-2012, Republic of Moldova, Europe
Printed at: see last page
ISBN: 978-620-8-35476-3

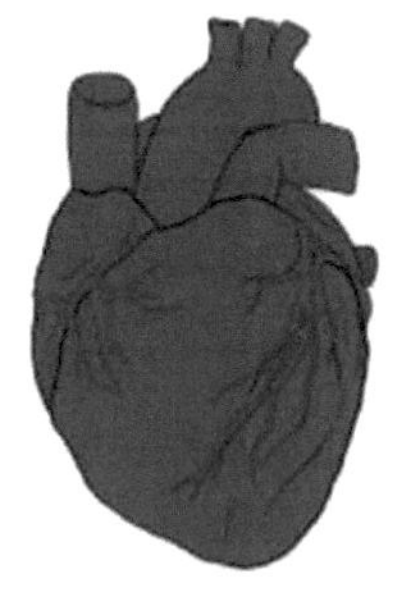

PROGNOSIS OF HEART FAILURE

IN SUB-SAHARAN AFRICA.

DR DOUNE NARCISSE

Cardiologist at CHU-RENAISSANCE

N'DJAMENA CHAD

DEDICACES

To ¡the Eternal my God,

Lord, you are my light. Were it not for your mercy and grace, I would be nothing. Thank you Lord for everything.

To my father BOZABE ZOUYANET Benjamin and my mother KYEBLOUABE PATALLE Tabitha

No words can express what you mean to me. You have always been there to guide me, advise me and support me. I will do my best to live up to your expectations. May God continue to bless you.

To my wife GARIA PATCHANNE, you have always been by my side in the most difficult times. I would like to express all my affection and gratitude.

To my children : EHKALBO DOUNE DAWI Wilfrid, DOUNE ADJOLBO Steeve and DOUNE AWONA Anaëlle, you are a gift from heaven to me. May GOD continue to bless and guide you.

To my brothers BEUNONE Davy and ANO Frédéric, our brotherhood is a sacred bond. You have spared no effort to contribute to my success. This work is yours.

To my aunt **TCHONFENE Catherine**, you are my second mother. Thank you for your support and your prayer.

ACKNOWLEDGEMENTS

Our Master Professor **Patrice ZABSONRE**, coordinator of the Diplôme d'Etudes Spécialisées (DES) in Cardiology at Joseph Ki-Zerbo University, Ouagadougou/Burkina Faso, and his team.

Table of contents

INTRODUCTION

With changing lifestyles, cardiovascular disease is becoming increasingly alarming, with heart failure the ultimate outcome. Heart failure (HF) is a frequent pathology, burdened with high morbidity and mortality. In recent years, its prevalence has been rising steadily worldwide. Two main factors explain this trend: the ageing of the population and the growing improvement in the management of cardiovascular diseases, the ultimate stage of which is heart failure [1]. Heart failure (HF) is associated with high mortality. Five-year survival is clearly inferior to that of certain cancers [2]. Assessment of prognostic factors can optimize management and reduce morbidity and mortality associated with heart failure, especially in resource-limited countries.

PROBLEM STATEMENT

In developed countries, the prevalence of CI is between 1% and 2% in the general population, reaching over 10% in patients aged over 70 [3]. Despite advances in the therapeutic management of CI, re-hospitalization remains frequent. The risk of re-hospitalization is estimated at 20% at 30 days, 30% at three months and 40% at one year, 70% of which can be avoided by management based on risk stratification [4].

In sub-Saharan Africa, heart failure is the leading cause of hospitalization in cardiology departments. Its in-hospital prevalence is 28.6% in Lomé, Togo, with an in-hospital mortality rate of 16.4% [5], 30% in Yaoundé, Cameroon, with an in-hospital mortality rate of 9.03% [6], and 14.44% in N'Djamena, Chad, with an in-hospital mortality rate of 18.3% [7].

In Burkina Faso, according to studies carried out in the cardiology department of the Centre Hospitalier Universitaire Yalgado Ouedraogo (CHU-YO), heart failure accounts for 42.9% of causes of hospitalization, with in-hospital mortality of 17.9% in 2014 [8], a high readmission rate, i.e. 36.8% of re-hospitalizations within the first year [9].

Despite considerable progress, which has given us a solid therapeutic arsenal, the morbidity and mortality of heart failure remain high. In France, it accounts for 200,000 hospitalizations and 22,000 deaths per year [1].

Prognostic assessment is a crucial step in the management of this disease, especially in our resource-constrained environment, in order to guide therapeutic decisions based on individual risk. It is therefore essential to have clinical, biological, electrocardiographic and echocardiographic parameters available for prognostic evaluation.

Most studies of heart failure in Burkina Faso and the sub-region have focused on epidemiological, clinical, therapeutic and evolutionary aspects. We therefore set out to study the adverse prognostic factors and stratify the risk of mortality in systolic heart failure in our context.

1. GENERAL

1.1 Definition and classification

1.1.1 Definition

According to TEuropean Society of Cardiology (ESC) 2016, heart failure (HF) is defined as a clinical syndrome characterized by chronic symptoms that may be accompanied by physical signs caused by a structural and/or functional cardiac abnormality, resulting in decreased cardiac output and/or increased intracardiac pressures at rest or during stress [3].

1.1.2 Classification

The new classification of CI (Table I) is based on the left ventricular ejection fraction (LVEF) [3] :

- ✓ Reduced LVEF CI (rLVEF CI), defined as LVEF < 40%,
- ✓ LVEF-preserved CI (LVEFpCI), defined as LVEF ≥ 50%,
- ✓ and IC with intermediate LVEF (ICFEi), defined as LVEF between 40% and 49%.

Systolic heart failure is the term used to describe heart failure with reduced LVEF and heart failure with intermediate LVEF.

Table I: Classification of heart failure [1].

IC type		ICFEr	ICFEi ICFEp	
	1	Symptoms ± physical signs of CI		
	2	LVEF < 40%	LVEF 40 - 49	LVEF ≥ 50%
Criteria	3	-	Elevated natriuretic peptide levels: BNP ≥ 35 pg/mL or NT-proBNP ≥ 125pg/mL At least one of the additional factors : A cardiac structural anomaly: LVH, OG dilatation (>34ml/m^2); Diastolic dysfunction: E/e'≥13 or e'< 9cm/s.	
Clinical signs may not be present in early-stage CHF (particularly in CHF-FEP) and in patients treated with diuretics.				

1.2 Pathophysiology

A-Heart failure with reduced ejection fraction

1.2.1 Impairment of systolic function [10,11].

The three determinants of systolic function that may be implicated in systolic function impairment are:

- ***Contractility***

Contractility or inotropism is the intrinsic capacity of a contractile unit to produce force.

Impaired contractility can be observed in dilated cardiomyopathy, myocarditis, dilated heart disease and almost all advanced heart disease.

- **Post-loading**

The afterload represents the force that the heart muscle must overcome to shorten itself. It is indirectly assessed by the resistance to left ventricular ejection. A pathologically significant increase in afterload leads to heart failure. This is the case in arterial hypertension, aortic stenosis and coarctation of the aorta.

- **Pre-loading**

According to Frank-Starling's law, after activation, a muscle fiber (myocardial or otherwise) develops a force proportional to its initial pre-activation length.

In the heart, this means that the fuller (distended) the ventricle, the greater the force developed during contractions. Preload is assessed indirectly by the filling volume of the ventricle (end-diastolic volume).

In pathology, increased preload can lead to heart failure. This is seen in mitral and aortic insufficiency.

1.2.2 Impaired diastolic function.

The three main determinants of diastolic function that can be implicated in this dysfunction are: relaxation, compliance and heart rate.

- **Relaxation**

Ventricular relaxation lowers protodiastolic intraventricular pressure below left atrial pressure, thus creating a genuine ventricular aspiration phenomenon: protodiastolic rapid ventricular filling. In pathology, relaxation may be slowed and/or incomplete in the case of altered energy metabolism in coronary insufficiency or left ventricular hypertrophy. As a result, filling is impeded and ventricular filling pressure rises, leading to diastolic heart failure. It is a physiological phenomenon that sets in with age, explaining the frequency of diastolic dysfunction in elderly subjects.

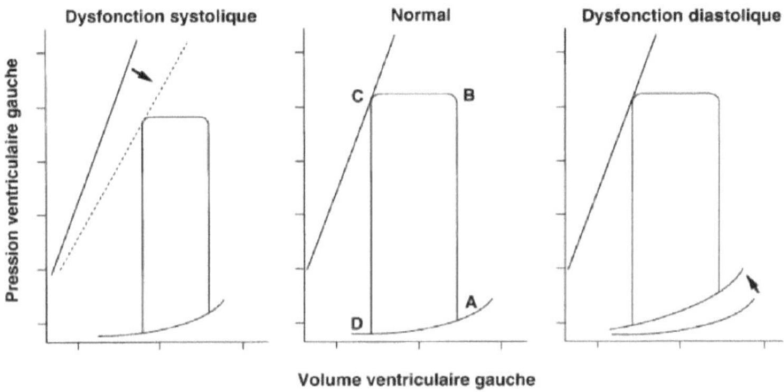

Figure 1: Pressure-volume curve: normal, systolic and diastolic dysfunction

- **Compliance**

Apart from any active phenomena, the ventricular wall exhibits a certain passive compliance linked to the elastic properties of the myocardium. Compliance is the relationship between the pressure in the ventricle and the volume of blood it contains. High compliance means the ventricle is easy to fill, while low compliance indicates a rigid ventricle. A decrease in compliance is accompanied by an increase in filling pressure, and consequently by a rise in left atrial and pulmonary pressures, responsible for dyspnea.

In pathology, myocardial fibrosis, sequelae of infarction and left ventricular wall hypertrophy may be responsible for this phenomenon. Chronic constrictive pericarditis represents a model of diastolic heart failure with pure compliance impairment and no impairment of myocardial function (and no impairment of ventricular relaxation).

- **Heart rate**

Heart rate increases at the expense of diastole. This results in a relaxation defect and a consequent increase in filling pressure, with repercussions upstream of the heart.

1.2.3 Compensating mechanisms

In response to impaired cardiac function, compensatory mechanisms are rapidly brought into play. These are of three types: cardiac, peripheral and neurohormonal [11].

- **Cardiac compensatory mechanisms**
  - ✓ Frank-Starling's Law:

According to this law, increased ventricular filling accentuates myocardial fiber stretch and enhances myocardial contraction. However, this is less effective than in normal subjects, as the intrinsic contractility of the myocardium is impaired and the increase in cardiac output is therefore limited. What's more, ventricular dilatation is accompanied by an increase in filling pressure, favoring the onset of congestive signs.

- ✓ Ventricular remodeling

It helps maintain systolic ejection volume. But this mechanism is energetically costly and deleterious over the long term.

- ✓ Sinus tachycardia

The increase in heart rate is dependent on sympathetic activation and allows a limited increase in cardiac output within a certain heart rate range, beyond which the shortening of filling time becomes deleterious in the medium term.

- **Peripheral compensatory mechanisms**
  - ✓ Redistribution of circulating blood flow

It is directed towards the "noble" organs: the cerebral and coronary circulations are favored over the cutaneous, renal, splanchnic and muscular-skeletal circulations, which are at the root of many symptoms.

✓ Hemoglobin facilitates oxygen release.

In heart failure, there is increased oxygen extraction, reflected in a rise in the arteriovenous oxygen difference. This extraction is linked to a decrease in the affinity of hemoglobin for oxygen.

➢ **Neurohormonal mechanisms**

✓ Vasoconstrictor Systems

- Sympathetic activation (noradrenalin): the drop in blood pressure recorded by baroreceptors located in the carotid sinuses and aortic arch generates afferent signals stimulating the cardioregulatory centers responsible for sympathetic stimulation. The aim of these systems is to maintain organ perfusion pressure by vasoconstricting and increasing blood volume.

- Renin-angiotensin-aldosterone system: angiotensin II is a powerful vasoconstrictor. It stimulates aldosterone secretion by the adrenal cortex, promotes cell proliferation and catecholamine release. The production of angiotensin II (from angiotensin I) is linked to plasma renin secretion in response either to a decrease in perfusion pressure in the afferent renal artery of the stretch-sensitive juxtaglomerular apparatus, or to direct stimulation of the juxtaglomerular apparatus by circulating catecholamines and the sympathetic nervous system, or to changes in the sodium load at the macula densa.

Angiotensin II secretion is cyclical and increases with each cardiac decompensation.

✓ Aldosterone:

It promotes sodium reabsorption and potassium loss (with risk of rhythm disorders). It is involved in myocardial fibrosis and cardiomyocyte remodeling.

1.2.4 Advanced heart failure

Heart failure inevitably progresses to advanced heart failure. The recommendations [12] and consensus conferences [13] of learned societies define patients with advanced heart failure according to the distinctive criteria listed in Table II.

Table II: Definition of advanced heart failure

ACC/AHA	Symptoms of heart failure at rest or with minimal activity. Full diagnostic work-up, including identification of comorbidity factors Maximum medical treatment
Consensus of American experts	Significant cardiac dysfunction Severe symptoms including dyspnea, asthenia, signs of low cardiac output at rest or with minimal activity Maximum medical treatment
ESC	Symptomatic patients remaining in NYHA stage IV Full diagnostic exploration Optimum medical treatment
ESC Heart Failure Association Working Group	Severe symptoms (NYHA III or IV) History of episodes of cardiac decompensation: fluid retention, low peripheral output. Severe cardiac dysfunction (at least one of the following signs): - LVEF < 30% - restrictive or pseudo-normal transmitral diastolic Doppler flow - increased ventricular filling pressures (LV and/or VD) - elevated BNP blood levels Severe impairment of exercise capacity (at least one of the following signs) - inability to make the slightest effort - six-minute walk test < 300 m - Peak VO2< 12 -14 ml/kg/min Hospitalization(s) for heart failure within the last six months. Optimal medical treatment.

1.2 Etiologies

As heart failure is the outcome of almost all cardiac diseases, etiological investigation is essential to detect any curable cause of heart failure. In our context, Doppler echocardiography is of invaluable help. The different etiologies of left and right heart failure according to the Collège des Enseignants de Cardiologie et Maladies Vasculaires [14] are summarized in Table III.

Table III: Main etiologies of heart failure

Etiologies of left-sided IC
- **Ischemic cardiomyopathy** - **Idiopathic dilated cardiomyopathy** - **Valvular cardiomyopathies: aortic stenosis, aortic insufficiency, mitral insufficiency, mitral stenosis** - **Hypertensive cardiomyopathy** - **Toxic heart disease: alcohol, chemotherapy, cocaine** - **Cardiac deficiency: avitaminosis B1 or beriberi** - **Obstructive and non-obstructive hypertrophic cardiomyopathy** - **Restrictive cardiomyopathy** - **Myocarditis: most often HIV viral** **-Overload cardiopathy: hemochromatosis and amyloidosis** **-Uncorrected congenital heart disease** - **Peripartum cardiomyopathy** - **Sarcoidosis, collagenoses, myopathies** - **Hyperoutput cardiac insufficiency: anemia, hyperthyroidism, arteriovenous fistula, Paget's disease, beriberi** - **Rhythmic cardiomyopathy**
Etiologies of right-sided CI
- **Pulmonary hypertension secondary to: left ventricular failure, mitral stenosis, chronic pulmonary pathology (pulmonary heart chronic), pulmonary embolism leading to acute pulmonary heart and/or chronicle** - **Pulmonary arterial hypertension usually primary, or associated with a connective tissue disease (scleroderma).** - **Congenital heart disease with left-right shunt: atrial septal defect, ventricular septal defect** - **Right-sided valve disease (rare)** - **Constrictive pericarditis, tamponade** - **Hyperflow IC** - **Right ventricular infarction** - **Arrhythmogenic right ventricular dysplasia**

1.4 DIAGNOSIS

1.4.1 Clinical diagnosis

The clinical diagnostic criteria for heart failure were grouped together using the Framingham cohort [15]. This study, initially based on cardiovascular risk factors, subsequently identified predictive factors for the development of heart failure. Criteria previously classified as "major" and "minor" are now grouped into "typical and less typical symptoms" and "specific and less specific signs". They are described in Table IV according to ESC 2016 [3].

Table IV: symptoms and clinical signs of heart failure according to ESC 2016

Symptoms	Clinical signs
Typical	**More specific**
Dyspnea **Orthopnea** **Paroxysmal nocturnal dyspnea** **Reduced exercise tolerance** **Fatigue, exhaustion, increased recovery time after exercise** **Swollen ankles**	**Increased jugular venous pressure** **Hepatojugular reflux** **Third heart sound (gallop rhythm)** **Peak shock deflection**
Less typical	**Less specific**
Nocturnal cough **Wheezing** **Feeling of fullness** **Loss of appetite** **Mental confusion (especially in the elderly)** **Depression** **Palpitations** **Dizziness, lightheadedness** **Syncope** **"Bendopnea" (bendopnea:dyspnea when the patient leans forward)**	**Weight gain (> 2 kg/week)** **Weight loss (advanced CI)** **Cachexia** **Heart murmur** **Peripheral edema (ankle, sacrum, scrotum)** **Pulmonary crackles** **Reduced air entry and dullness at lung bases (pleural effusion)** **Tachycardia** **Irregular pulse** **Tachypnea** **Cheyne-Stokes breathing** **Hepatomegaly** **Ascites** **Cold ends** **Oliguria, drop in pulse pressure.**

There are no symptoms or clinical signs to confirm or exclude the diagnosis [16]. Biological markers (BNP or NT-proBNP) and cardiac

Doppler ultrasound are necessary to confirm the diagnosis. A
he algorithm for diagnosing CI in non-acute situations is shown in figure2.

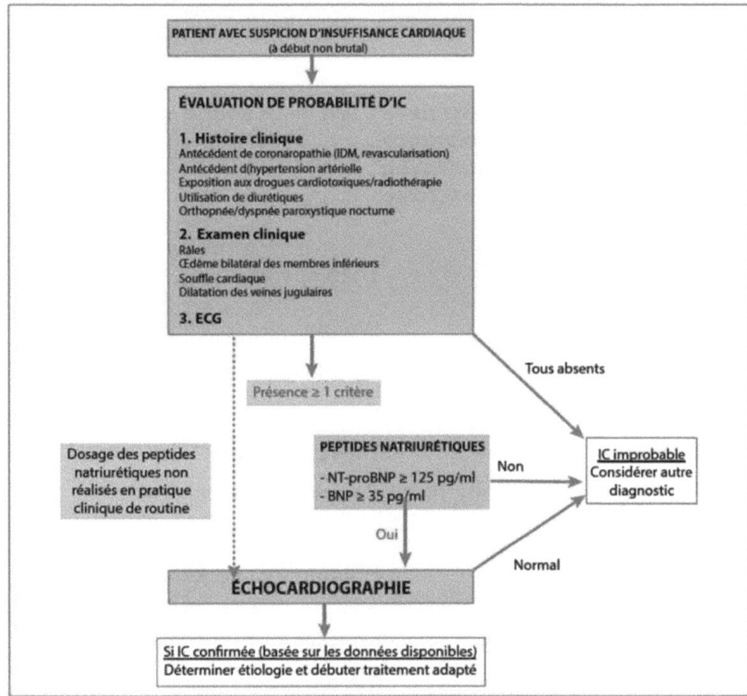

Figure 2: Diagnostic scheme for the diagnosis of heart failure with a non-abrupt onset.

BNP = B-type natriuretic peptide; ECG = electrocardiogram; HF = heart failure; NT-proBNP = N-terminal pro-B-type natriuretic peptide.

1.4.2 Paraclinical examinations

a- Determination of natriuretic peptides [17,18].

BNP and NT-pro BNP are not specific markers of CI. The use of natriuretic peptides (NP) is recommended to rule out CI. However, they are not diagnostic. Other comorbidities or particular physiological situations may lead to NP secretion: NP values increase with age, renal failure, pulmonary embolism, chronic pulmonary heart disease, arterial hypertension, pulmonary arterial hypertension, acute or chronic ischemia, valvulopathy and left ventricular hypertrophy. NP levels fall after initiation of symptomatic diuretic treatment of CHF, which reduces the sensitivity of this test after initiation of treatment.

b- Doppler echocardiography

The diagnosis, suspected clinically or biologically (BNP), must be confirmed by objective evidence of cardiac dysfunction at rest, whether structural or functional, thanks to Doppler echocardiography, which calculates the left ventricular ejection fraction (LVEF) and measures the size of the left ventricle (LV), parietal thickness, study the condition of the heart valves, look for pulmonary arterial hypertension (PAH) and assess the quality of left ventricular ejection and filling.

Echocardiography is used to determine the type of CI. (Table I)

c- Electrocardiogram (ECG)

It is rarely normal. An abnormal ECG increases the probability of a diagnosis of CHF, but has low specificity. Certain ECG abnormalities can provide information on the etiology. It can reveal :

- ✓ most often sinus tachycardia,
- ✓ complete atrial fibrillation arrhythmia (CAFA) or atrial flutter,
- ✓ signs of left ventricular overload,
- ✓ complete or incomplete left bundle branch block,
- ✓ sequelae of necrosis,
- ✓ sometimes ventricular extrasystole, which has a negative prognostic effect (myocardial failure).

d- Chest X-ray

It is useful for looking for signs compatible with heart failure, such as cardiomegaly and signs of pleuropulmonary repercussions, but above all for ruling out a pulmonary etiology for the symptomatology. Other tests to be performed on patients with heart failure [19] are shown in Table V.

Table V: Tests to be carried out on patients diagnosed with heart failure

Investigations to be considered in all patients diagnosed with CI
Laboratory **Complete blood count** **Sodium, potassium, calcium, urea, creatinine, creatinine clearance (CKD-)** **Epi)** **Liver enzymes, bilirubin** **Glycated haemoglobin** **Lipid profile** **TSH** **Ferritin, iron saturation level** **Natriuretic peptides** **Other biological tests may be carried out depending on the clinical suspicion of a suspected pathology (e.g. Lyme serology, HIV, etc.).**
Exercise test **Recommended for heart transplant assessment (cardiopulmonary exercise test)** **To identify the cause of unexplained dyspnea** **To optimize the prescription for cardiac training**
Right heart catheterization **Is recommended in cases of severe IC with a view to transplantation**

The ESC recommends more advanced tests such as stress echocardiography, MRI and cardiac catheterization, depending on the patient's profile and clinical presentation. These indications should be discussed with the cardiologist. Certain tests are not feasible in our setting, due to the limited technical resources available, reducing the diagnosis of heart failure to the clinic and echocardiography.

1.3 TREATMENT

1.5.1 Treatment of heart failure with reduced LVEF (rLVEF)

➢ **Treatment objectives**

According to the ESC 2016 recommendations on the diagnosis and treatment of heart failure, the main treatment goals are [3]:

- ✓ improved clinical condition, functional capacity and quality of life,
- ✓ preventing hospitalization,
- ✓ and reduced mortality.

➢ **Principles of treatment**

The main principles of rEFEI treatment, based on pathophysiological knowledge, consist of :

- ✓ treat the cause if possible,
- ✓ combat fluid retention,
- ✓ reduce afterload and preload,
- ✓ improve myocardial contractility,
- ✓ reduce cardiac workload,
- ✓ increase cardiac output,
- ✓ prevent rhythmic complications,
- ✓ treat the triggering factor and prevent thromboembolic complications.

➢ **Therapeutic methods**

A- Non-medicinal means: therapeutic education and hygienic-dietary measures.

Patients with heart failure should receive therapeutic education, which consists in explaining to them and their families the disease, the factors that may aggravate it, the mechanism of action of the medication, the importance of taking the medication regularly, the benefits of non-pharmacological measures and regular weight monitoring.

Hygienic and dietary measures should include: sodium restriction, water restriction (1.5 L per day) in the event of a flare-up or signs of congestion, weight monitoring, smoking cessation and influenza vaccination.
Cardiovascular exercise rehabilitation should be undertaken in patients with stable heart failure. The simplest method is the six-minute test. It should be carried out before discharge from hospital.

B- Medication.

Today, the treatment of chronic heart failure with impaired LVEF is based on sound recommendations derived from multiple therapeutic trials. However, the treatment of CHF with preserved EF remains much less codified.

1- **Converting enzyme inhibitors (CEIs).**

ACE inhibitors now represent the cornerstone of medical treatment for heart failure, based on randomized studies since CONSENSUS [34]. They are recommended as first-line therapy, in combination with a beta-blocker, in all symptomatic and non-symptomatic patients with reduced LVEF, to reduce the risk of hospitalization for heart failure and premature death [34,35]. They can be replaced by an ARB2 in case of side effects. Dosage should be gradually increased in two-week increments, as long as systolic blood pressure remains above 90 mmHg, in the absence of orthostatic hypotension.

2- **Angiotensin 2 receptor antagonists (ARB2).**

ARB2s are recommended to reduce the risk of IC hospitalization and premature death in patients with reduced LVEF who cannot tolerate an ACE inhibitor because of cough. These patients should also receive a beta-blocker and a corticosteroid mineral receptor antagonist (MRA) [3,36].

3- Beta-blockers

The use of beta-blockers in heart failure has been revolutionary over the past two decades. Previously, they were contraindicated in heart failure because of their negative inotropic effect. Clinical studies have amply demonstrated the improvement in symptoms, exercise tolerance and ventricular function in heart failure under long-term beta-blocker therapy. These include the CIBIS II study with bisoprolol (DETENSIEL), which impressively confirmed the reduction in mortality [37], and the MERIT HF study with metoprolol (SELOKEN) [38]. Both studies had to be terminated prematurely after one year, due to positive results with active treatment. Beta-blockers are currently indicated in combination in systolic heart failure to reduce the rate of rehospitalization and early mortality (class I recommendation, level of evidence A).

Beta-blockers are introduced outside the period of decompensation, at a low dose and titrated progressively until the effective, tolerated dose is reached.

4- Diuretics

Although diuretics have not been shown to reduce mortality or hospitalization, they relieve dyspnea and edema and are an essential treatment for systolic heart failure (class I recommendation, level of evidence B) [3]. The aim is to use the minimum dose necessary to restore and maintain euvolemia ("dry weight").

5- Mineralocorticoid receptor antagonists (MRAs)

An MRA (spironolactone or eplerenone) is recommended as second-line therapy in all patients who remain symptomatic with LVEF less than or equal to 35% on treatment with an ACE inhibitor/ARB2 and a beta-blocker to reduce the risk of hospitalization for IC and premature death [39] (class I recommendation, level of evidence A) [3]. MRAs should be used with caution in patients with severe renal impairment whose GFR is less than or equal to 30 ml/min and whose kalemia is greater than 5 mmol/l.

6- Ivabradine

Ivabradine is an inhibitor of sinus node If channels. Its effect is to slow heart rate in sinus rhythm. It has no effect on ventricular rate in cases of complete atrial fibrillation arrhythmia. It is indicated in patients with an LVEF of less than 35%, in sinus rhythm whose heart rate is greater than or equal to 70 beats per minute and who remain symptomatic despite treatment with a combination of beta-blockers, ACE inhibitors or ARBs and MRAs [40] (class IIa recommendation, level of evidence B).

7- Digoxin

Digoxin is increasingly losing its place in the treatment of heart failure. Unlike ivabradine, digoxin does not reduce mortality and may have ventricular arrhythmogenic effects [41]. It reduces the risk of hospitalization in patients with an LVEF below 35% who remain symptomatic (NYHA class II-III) despite treatment with a beta-blocker, an ACE inhibitor (or ARB2) and an MRA (class IIb recommendation, level of evidence B) [3]. Digoxin may be considered in patients with atrial fibrillation, when ventricular rate remains too high (above 110 bpm) or when beta-blockers are poorly tolerated or contraindicated (class IIa recommendation, level of evidence B) [3]. Dosage is adapted to renal function.

8- Angiotensin-neprilysin receptor blocker

The angiotensin-neprilysin receptor blocker (ANRB) is a new therapeutic class appearing as a third-line treatment for symptomatic patients, in the form of a combination of sacubitril (a selective neprilysin inhibitor)/valsartan (ARB2) [3]. Not available in our pharmacies, this compound combines the effects of neprilysin inhibition (a neutral endopeptidase responsible for the degradation of natriuretic peptides exerting an antifibrotic effect), and antiproliferative effects reducing left ventricular hypertrophy. This favors cardiac relaxation, stimulates diuresis and natriuresis, and promotes vasodilation [42], as well as angiotensin 2 ATI receptor vasodilation. This treatment is recommended as an alternative to ACE inhibitors to reduce the risk of hospitalization for CHF and death in ambulatory patients with reduced LVEF who remain symptomatic despite optimal treatment with ACE inhibitors, beta-blockers and MRAs (class I recommendation, level of evidence B) [3].

9- Hydralazine and isosorbide dinitrate

This combination should be considered as an alternative in well-identified patients with LVEF less than or equal to 35%, or with LVEF less than 45% associated with dilated cardiomyopathy in NYHA functional class III-IV, despite treatment with ACE inhibitors, beta-blockers and MRAs (mineralocorticoid receptor antagonists) to reduce the risk of hospitalization for IC and death [43]. (class IIa recommendation, level of evidence B). This combination may be considered in symptomatic patients with reduced LVEF who cannot tolerate either ACE inhibitors or ARB2 to reduce the risk of death (class IIb recommendation, level of evidence B)[3].

C- Instrumental and surgical resources.

S **The automatic implantable defibrillator**

For secondary prevention, implantation of an implantable automatic defibrillator (ICD) is indicated in patients with a ventricular rhythm disorder responsible for hemodynamic instability, with a functional life expectancy of more than one year, to reduce the risk of sudden death [17] (class I recommendation, level of evidence A) [3].

S **Cardiac resynchronization**

Multicenter studies have clearly demonstrated the benefit in terms of morbidity and mortality of biventricular resynchronization in selected patients [44,45]. In around 70% of patients, resynchronization provides a significant benefit in terms of :

- functional signs, quality of life and quality of exercise,
- of cardiac function and ventricular remodelling,
- morbidity and mortality. In fact, resynchronization reduces the number of hospitalizations for cardiac decompensation and the number of days spent in hospital.

J **heart transplantation**

Heart transplantation is a recognized treatment for end-stage heart failure for which there is no other therapeutic alternative. It is the only chance of survival. Despite the absence of randomized studies, it is considered to significantly increase survival (76% at one year and 67% at five years), exercise capacity, return to work and quality of life compared with conventional treatment [46].

1.5.2 Treatment of heart failure with preserved LVEF (pLVEF)

It is not yet well codified, as guidelines recognize that no treatment has yet demonstrated a benefit in terms of morbidity and mortality. Diuretics are used to control symptoms of fluid retention. Appropriate management of hypertension or ischemic heart disease, as well as ventricular rhythm control, is also recommended in ACFA. A small study has demonstrated the benefit of a calcium channel blocker, verapamil, in this indication [47].

1.4 Prognosis

1.6.1 Mortality in heart failure.

The prognosis of heart failure is poor in the absence of a curable cause; 50% of patients die within four years. Forty percent of patients admitted to hospital with heart failure die or are readmitted within one year [20].

The number of heart failure deaths has risen despite advances in treatment. This is due to an increase in the prevalence of heart failure patients, linked to better management of ischemic heart disease and hypertension. Heart failure mainly affects the elderly. The aging of the population also contributes to the growing incidence of heart failure [21]. Mortality in heart failure patients was one to three times higher than in control subjects of the same age [15]. According to the National Heart, Lung

and Blood Institute", the death rates at 30^{e} day, one year and five years after hospitalization for heart failure were 10.4%, 22% and 42.3% respectively [22]. Blacks had a higher five-year mortality rate than whites ($p<0.05$).

1.6.2 Prognostic factors

1- Non-modifiable risk factors

- ✓ age: older age is associated with higher mortality in the majority of studies [23].
- ✓ gender: several studies have identified male gender as an unfavorable prognostic factor [24].

2- Modifiable risk factors

- ✓ diabetes: it has been shown that diabetes is associated with a poor prognosis, whether type I or type II [25].
- ✓ For other risk factors (hypertension, smoking, dyslipidemia), the results of survival studies are discordant [26].
- ✓ Clinical prognostic factors
- ✓ Etiology: the ischemic origin of heart failure has been described as a powerful poor prognostic factor [27].
- ✓ Comorbidities: the presence of cardiovascular comorbidities, such as stroke, renal failure or lung disease, is associated with a poor prognosis [28].

- ✓ Elevated heart rate, lower-limb oedema and crepitus rales are associated with high mortality [23, 28].

3- Biological prognostic factors :

- ✓ Hyponatremia: hyponatremia is associated with higher mortality, irrespective of the use and dose of diuretics used [29].
- ✓ An increase in creatinine or a decrease in glomerular filtration rate are also poor prognostic factors [30].
- ✓ Anemia, which aggravates the peripheral tissue oxygenation defect, is associated with a poor prognosis [29].

4- Electrocardiographic prognostic factors: atrial fibrillation, left bundle branch block and ventricular tachycardia are associated with higher mortality in patients with heart failure [23, 24, 31].

5- Echocardiographic prognostic factors: impaired left ventricular ejection fraction (LVEF), increased systolic pulmonary artery pressure (SPAP), increased left ventricular end-diastolic diameter (LVEDD), right ventricular dysfunction and mitral regurgitation are associated with high mortality [32, 33].

2 OUR STUDY

2.1 Conceptual framework

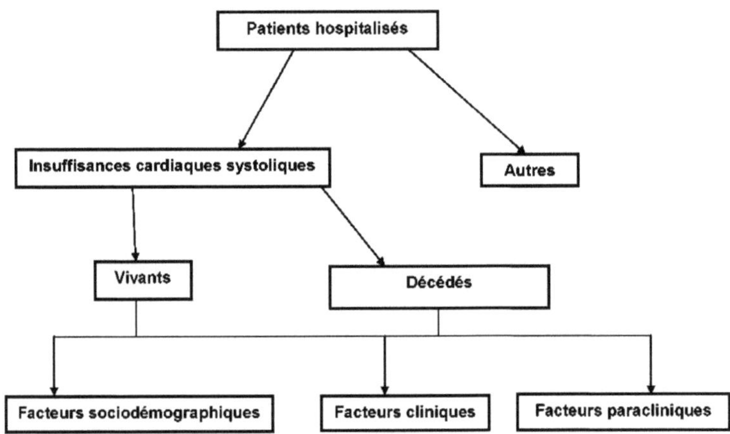

Figure 3: conceptual framework

2.2 RESEARCH QUESTION

What are the clinical and biological factors associated with mortality in systolic heart failure?

2.3 OBJECTIVES

➢ ***General objective***

To study the factors associated with inpatient systolic heart failure mortality in the cardiology department of CHU-YO from January 1er 2017 to December 31 2018.

➢ **Specific objectives**

1- To identify sociodemographic factors associated with mortality in systolic heart failure in the cardiology department of

CHUYO ;

2- To identify the clinical factors associated with mortality in systolic heart failure in the cardiology department of CHU-YO ;

3- Identify paraclinical factors associated with mortality in systolic heart failure in the cardiology department of CHU-YO.

2.4 METHODOLOGY

2.4.1 Type of study

This was a retrospective, case-control study.

2.4.2 Study framework

The study took place in the cardiology ward of the Yalgado Ouédraogo University Hospital. The cardiology unit is part of the Department of Medicine and Medical Specialties.

➢ **Premises and equipment**

The cardiology department at CHU-YO includes:

- the outpatient, follow-up and functional exploration unit. It includes doctors' offices for outpatient consultations and non-invasive explorations for both inpatients and outpatients;
- the cardiac stimulation and electrophysiology unit (not yet operational), located in the main trauma emergency building;
- the inpatient unit comprises six (06) hospital wards with a total capacity of 26 beds, including two wards with two beds each for the first category, two wards with three beds each for the second category and two wards with eight beds each for the third category;
- the cardiac intensive care unit (USIC) has four beds and is equipped with scopes, an emergency cart and a defibrillator;
- an on-call room for nursing staff;
- a treatment room;
- a 50-seat meeting room;
- a doctor's room ;

- a room for the care unit supervisor;
- a room for support staff ;
- a store.

➢ **Our staff**

The cardiology department is staffed by eight cardiologists, including one full professor, one associate professor, three assistant professors of cardiology and three practicing cardiologists. These doctors are assisted in their care, research and teaching activities by forty doctors enrolled on the Diplôme d'Etudes Spécialisées in cardiology, twelve nurses, six ward attendants and five stretcher-bearers.

Table VI: Inpatient activity report 2018

pathology	Prevalence (%)	Mortality (%)
Heart failure	**252 (38,3%)**	**33(40%)**
VTE	157(23,9%)	11(13,4%)
Hypertensive emergencies	87(13,22%)	15(18%)
Valvulopathy	53(8,06%)	10(12%)
Acute coronary syndrome	41 (6,23%)	4(5%)
Pericarditis	25(3,8%)	3(3,6%)
Endocarditis	8(1,21%)	1(1%)
Other	35(5,32%)	6(7%)
Total	658 (100%)	83(100%)

Others: BAV, CPC, AVK accidents, aortic dissection, etc.

2.4.3 Study period

Our study covered the period from January 1, 2017 to December 31, 2018, i.e. two years.

2.4.4 Study population

a- Inclusion criteria

- ✓ **For cases,** we included the clinical records of patients over 15 years of age hospitalized for systolic heart failure (presenting clinical signs of IC at admission and Doppler echocardiographic evidence of systolic dysfunction) who died during hospitalization.
- ✓ **For controls**, clinical records were included for patients over 15 years of age hospitalized for systolic heart failure (clinically presenting signs of IC at admission and Doppler echocardiography showing elements of systolic dysfunction) who were discharged alive.

b- Exclusion criteria

Clinical records of patients (cases and controls) with Doppler echocardiograms that could not be used to complete the survey form were excluded.

2.4.5 Sampling

$$N \geq \frac{P(1-P)(1+\frac{1}{c})(z\alpha+z\beta)^2}{(P0-P1)^2} \qquad P=\frac{P1+c\times P0}{1+c}$$

Cas = 26, Témoins = 26 × 2 = 52

N≥ 78. *N= la taille de l'échantillon,*

N= 162 files collected (Cases: 54, controls: 108, i.e. two controls for one case)

C= number of controls per case: For our study c= 2 (two controls for one case) p = proportion of cases exposed (prevalence of anemia in patients dying of heart failure (39% [48]),

Po= proportion of exposed controls (prevalence of anemia in living heart failure patients: 6% [48])

Zα= the value of Z for the first-species risk (for α= 5%, Za= 1.96)

Zβ= the Z value for 1-β power (for 80% power, β= 20% and Zβ= 0.84).

2.4.3 Data collection

Data were collected using a self-designed data collection form. The parameters studied were epidemiological, clinical and paraclinical (biological, electrocardiographic and echocardiographic).

- ✓ **Epidemiological data** included: age, gender, occupation.
- ✓ **Clinical data**
    - History of CI
    - cardiovascular risk factors: age, hypertension, diabetes, smoking, dyslipidemia, obesity
    - co-morbidities (renal failure, lung disease, anemia, stroke, pulmonary embolism),
    - NYHA dyspnea stage,
    - blood pressure,
    - heart rate,

- the sound of a left gallop,
- signs of DCI
- the etiology of CI,

✓ **Paraclinical data**

They included :

1- Biology:

- Rhesus blood group,
- Glycemia,
- Creatinine,
- Urea,
- Uric acid,
- Hemoglobin level,
- Natremia,
- Kalemia,
- Total cholesterol,
- LDL,
- Triglycerides.

2- Electrocardiogram

- Heart rate,
- TDR : ESV, ACFA, TV
- TDC: BAV, BBD, BBG,

3- Doppler echocardiography

a- Left ventricular parameters

- DTDVG,
- DTSVG,
- SIV thickness,
- PP thickness,
- Indexed VG mass,

- FE (using the TEICHOLZ method),
- FE (SIMPSON method),
- OG diameter,
- Surface OG,
- Volume OG,
- Functional IM,
- E/A ratio (LV filling pressure).

b- Right ventricle parameters

- Diameter VD,
- TAPSE,
- Surface OD,
- PAPS.

✓ **Therapeutic aspects**

Drug therapy: beta blockers, ACE inhibitors, ARB2, loop diuretics, anti-aldosterone, vasodilators, antiplatelet agents, anti-Vitamin K, tonicardiac drugs, statins, amiodarone.

2.4.4 Operational definitions of variables

➢ **Epidemiological**

Age (FDRCV): FDRCV is defined as age greater than or equal to 45 in men and greater than or equal to 55 in women.

➢ **Clinics**

Systolic heart failure was defined by the presence of signs of heart failure associated with less than 50% impairment of left ventricular systolic function on transthoracic Doppler echocardiography.

Clinical **right heart failure** was defined by the presence of exertional hepatalgia, lower limb edema or congestive hepatomegaly.

The severity of heart failure was judged by the functional stage of the

New York Heart Association (NYHA) Classification:

- ✓ Stage I: no symptoms or limitation of ordinary physical activity;
- ✓ Stage II: modest limitation of physical activity: comfortable at rest, but ordinary activity causes fatigue, palpitations, dyspnea;
- ✓ Stage III: marked reduction in physical activity: comfortable at rest, but less physical activity than usual causes symptoms and objective signs of cardiac dysfunction;
- ✓ Stage IV: severe limitation: symptoms present even at rest.

Cardiovascular risk factors

- Hypertensive: known hypertensive patient, documented and recorded in the clinical record,
- Diabetic: diabetic patient documented and recorded in the clinical record,
- Tobacco: active or weaned smoking for less than three years recorded in the clinical record

Comorbidities

- Anemia when hemoglobin < 13g/dl in men and 12g/dl in women,
- Renal insufficiency when creatinine clearance < 60/min calculated according to the CKD-EPI formula,
- Hyponatremia when natraemia < 135 mmol/l,
- Hypokalemia when kalemia < 3.5 mmol/l,

➢ **Echocardiographic parameter standards**

S **Left ventricular systolic function** [3].

Left ventricular ejection fraction (LVEF): 63 ± 6%. Based on the LVEF value, we defined a :

- Left ventricular systolic function preserved if LVEF ≥ 50% ;
- intermediate left ventricular systolic function if LVEF= 40 - 49% ;

- reduced left ventricular systolic function if LVEF < 40%; left ventricular shortening fraction: 36 ± 6%.

Other echocardiographic parameters

- ✓ Dilated left ventricle if telediastolic diameter > 56 mm ;
- ✓ High filling pressure if E/A ≥ 2 ;
- ✓ Dilated OG if diameter > 40 mm and surface area ≥ 20cm^2 ;
- ✓ Dilated VD if telediastolic diameter > 23 mm ;
- ✓ OD dilated if surface > 14 cm ,^{2}
- ✓ Impaired VD systolic function if TAPSE < 16 mm ;
- ✓ PAH if PAPS greater than 30 mm Hg before age 50 and PAPS greater than 40 mm Hg after age 50 ;
- ✓ Arterial hypotension if systolic blood pressure (SBP) < 90 mm Hg ;
- ✓ Hypertension if SAP ≥ 140 mm Hg and/or DBP ≥ 90 mm Hg ;
- ✓ Hypoglycemia if fasting blood glucose < 4 mmol/L ;

Normal glomerular filtration rate (GFR) if > 90 ml/min.

- mild renal insufficiency if GFR 60 - 90 ml/min ;
- moderate renal insufficiency if GFR 30 - 50 ml/min ;
- severe renal failure if GFR 15 - 29 ml/min ;
- end-stage renal failure if GFR < 15ml/min.

2.4.5 Data capture and analysis

The data collected was recorded on a computer, using EPI data and Microsoft 2010 software. Statistical analysis was carried out using STATA 15 software. As part of the selection of independent variables, we performed bivariate analyses using appropriate tests (chi2) to analyze associations and determine the variables to be included in the stepwise regression model (Roc curve), with a significance level of 5%. We then carried out a multivariate analysis.

2.4.6 Ethical considerations

The coding form is anonymous and includes the patient's file number as an identity reference.

2.5 RESULTS

In our study, we recorded 54 patients who died during hospitalization for systolic heart failure (cases) and 108 patients hospitalized for heart failure and discharged alive (controls), i.e. one case for every two controls. During the same period, 1,512 patients were hospitalized, broken down by pathology as follows:

- ✓ Heart failure: 569 (37.6%),
- ✓ Venous thromboembolic disease: 354 (23.4%),
- ✓ Hypertensive emergencies: 184 (12.16%),
- ✓ Valvulopathy: 124 (8.20%),
- ✓ Acute coronary syndrome: 90 (5.9%),
- ✓ Pericarditis: 55 (3.6%),
- ✓ CPC: 30 (2%),
- ✓ Endocarditis: 21 (1.38%),
- ✓ Other: 85.

2.5.1 Bivariate analysis of socio-demographic factors

- **Patient distribution by age group**

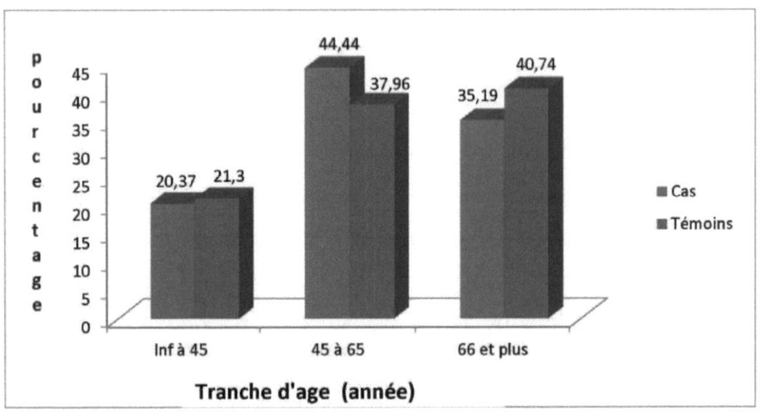

Figure 4: Age distribution

Mortality was highest in the 45 to 65 age group (44%). Bivariate analysis showed that there was no association between age and mortality (p= 0.71).

The mean age of all patients was : 58.24 ± 1.36 years and a 95% confidence interval [55.24 - 60.93]. The mean age of cases was 57.38 ± 2.3 years and that of controls 58.66 ± 1.68 years.

- **Patient distribution by gender**

In our study population, the proportion of males among cases was higher than that of controls, with a sex ratio of 1.7 in cases and 1.4 in controls. Bivariate analysis concluded that gender was not associated with mortality (p= 0.57). Figure 1 shows the gender distribution of cases and controls.

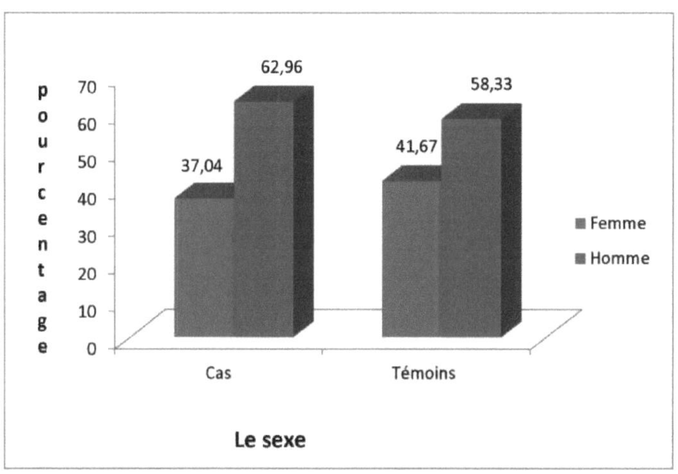

Figure 5: Gender distribution of cases and controls

➢ **Distribution of patients by old and new cases of heart failure**

Table VI: Distribution by history of heart failure

Former CI case	Case	Witnesses	OR
No	15 (27,78%)	44 (40,74%)	1
Yes	**39 (72,22%)**	**64 (59,26%)**	**3,78**
Total	54 (100%)	108 (100%)	

P=0,000

According to this table, previous heart failure was more frequent in our study population, with 72% of cases and 59% of controls. In univariate analysis (**p= 0.000** and **OR= 3.78)**, we noted that long-standing heart failure represented a risk factor for heart failure mortality compared with patients hospitalized for the first time for heart failure.

➢ **Distribution of patients by duration of CI evolution**

Table VII: Distribution by duration of CI evolution

CI duration	Case	Witnesses	Odds ratio
Under months	15 (27,78%)	64 (59,26%)	1
1 - 12 months	8 (14,81%)	14 (12,96%)	**2,43**
13 - 24 months	13 (24,04%)	13 (12,04%)	**4,26**
Over 25 months	18 (33,33%)	17 (15,74%)	**4,51**
Total	54 (100%)	108 (100%)	**P=0,001**

The mean overall duration of heart failure was 13.6 ± 1.6 months. The mean duration for **cases was 21.3± 3.2 months**. It was **9.7± 1.3**

months for controls. According to the table above, the duration of heart failure was strongly associated with mortality (**p=0.001)**.
The risk of mortality increased with the duration of heart failure (**OR=4.5** when heart failure had progressed for more than 25 months).

➢ **Breakdown by length of hospital stay**

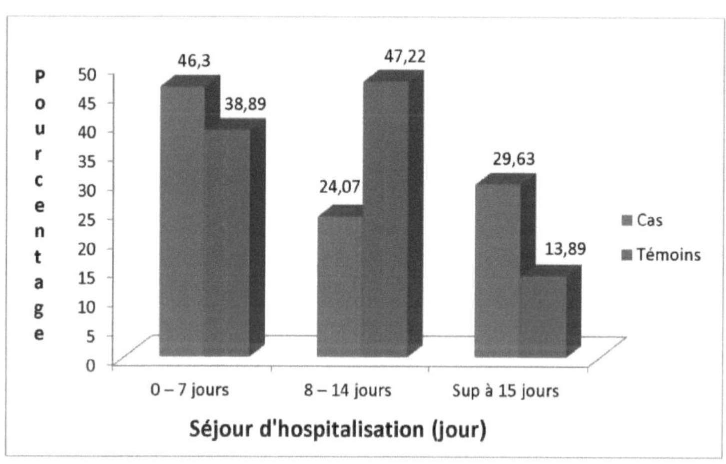

Figure 6: Breakdown by length of hospital stay

The mean length of stay for our study population was 10.2 ± 0.5 days. Cases had an average stay of 11.5 ± 1.2 days. Controls had an average stay of 9.6 ± 0.5 days.

According to the analysis, length of hospital stay was associated with mortality (p= 0.007). Most patients (46.3%) died within the first week of hospitalization. In contrast, most controls (47.22%) were discharged during the second week.

- **Summary of socio-demographic factors associated with mortality**

The socio-demographic factors associated with mortality were: previous heart failure, age of heart failure and length of hospital stay. These factors are summarized in the table below.

Table VIII: Summary table of socio-demographic factors associated with mortality

independent variable	Cases (%)	Controls (%)	p-value	Odd ratio
History of CHF				
No	15 (27,78%)	44 (40,74%)		
Yes	39 (72,22%)	64 (59,26%)	**0,000**	**3,78**
IC seniority				
Inf in Imois	15 (27,78%)	64 (59,26%)		
1 - 12 months	8 (14,81%)	14 (12,96%)	0,091	2,4
13 - 24 months	13 (24,04%)	13 (12,04%)	**0,003**	**4,25**
Over 25 months	18 (33,33%)	17 (15,74%)	**0,001**	**4,51**
Stay				
0 - 7 days	25 (46,30%)	42 (38,89%)		
8 - 14 days	13 (24,07%)	51 (47,22%)		
More than 15 days	16 (29,63%)	15 (13,89%)	**0,007**	**1,79**

2.5.2 Bivariate analysis of clinical factors

- **Distribution of patients according to the presence of risk factors cardiovascular**

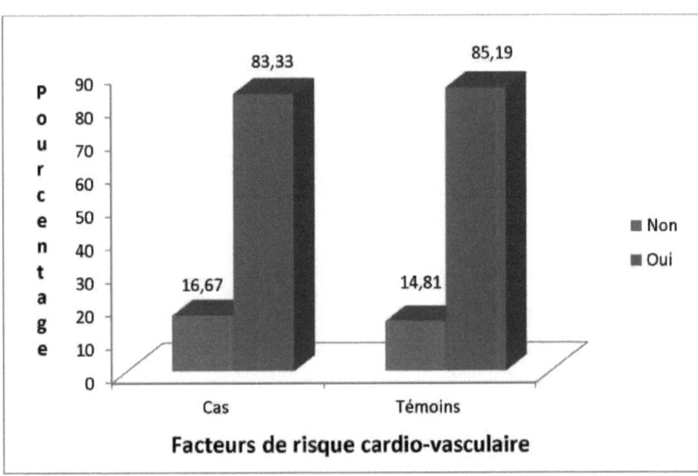

Figure 3: Distribution of cases and controls according to the presence of FDRCV in cases and controls

According to this figure, over 80% of patients had a cardiovascular risk factor (83.33% in cases and 85.19% in controls). In univariate analysis, the presence of cardiovascular risk factors was not associated with mortality (p=0.75).

- **Distribution of patients by dyspnea stage**

Almost all cases (92.59%) were admitted with NYHA stage III and IV dyspnea. More than half the controls were admitted with NYHA stage III dyspnea. In univariate analysis, there was an association between dyspnea stage and mortality (p= 0.004). This is illustrated in the figure below.

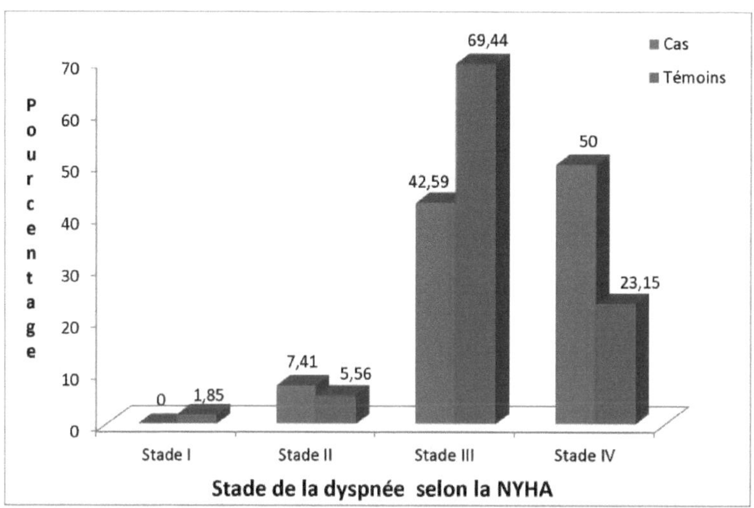

Figure 4: Dyspnea stage distribution

- **Distribution by systolic blood pressure**

Table IX: Distribution by PAS

PAS (mm Hg)	Case	Witnesses	p	OR	IC
0 à 90	**30 (55,56%)**	**16 (14,81%)**	**0,000**	**6,607**	**3,03 - 14,36**
91 à 139	21 (38,89%)	74 (68,52%)		1	
140 and more	3 (5,56%)	18 (16,67%)	0,428	0,58	0,15 - 2,18
Total	54 (100%)	108 (100%)			

According to this table, arterial hypotension was strongly associated with mortality (**p= 0.000, OR= 6.60**). Systolic hypertension, on the other hand, was not associated with mortality (p= 0.428).

Overall mean systolic blood pressure was **106.6 ± 2.1 mmHg**. It was **80** ± 4.4 **mmHg** for cases and **115.4** ± 1.8 **mmHg** for controls.

- **Distribution of patients by diastolic blood pressure**

Table X: Distribution by PAD

PAD (mm Hg)	Case	Witnesses	OR	p	IC
0 à 59	**18 (33,33%)**	**4 (3,70%)**	**10,4**	**0,000**	**3,29 - 33,20**
60 à 89	**34 (62,96%)**	**79 (73,15%)**	**1**		
90 and over	**2 (3,70%)**	**25 (23,15%)**	**0,18**	**0,027**	**0,04 - 0,82**
Total	**54 (100%)**	**108 (100%)**			

The above table shows that low diastolic blood pressure was strongly associated with mortality (**p=0.000 OR= 10.4**). The mean diastolic blood pressure of all patients was **69 ± 1.6mmHg**. It was **54.4± 3.2mmHg** for cases and **76.4 ±** 1.**3mmHg** for controls.

- **Distribution by heart rate**

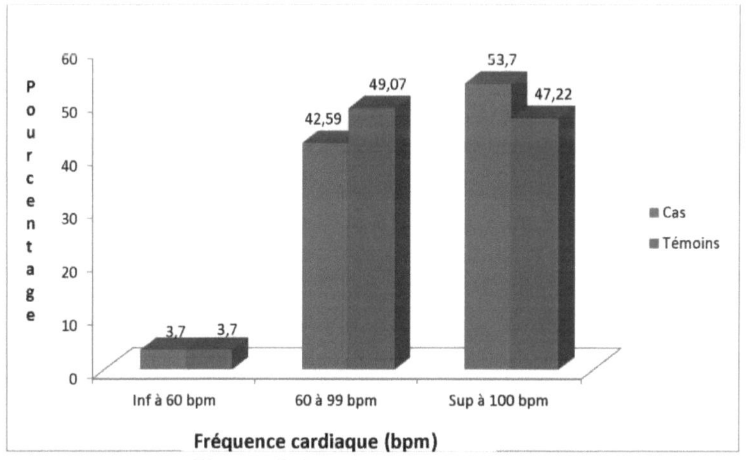

Figure 5: Distribution by heart rate

The mean heart rate for all patients was 99.8 ± 1.8 bpm. It was 100.2 ± 3.5 bpm for cases and 99.7 ± 2 bpm for controls.

According to the analysis, tachycardia or bradycardia was not associated with mortality ($p = 0.7$).

➢ Summary of clinical factors associated with mortality

Table XI: Summary table of clinical factors associated with mortality

Independent variable	Cases (%)	Controls (%)	p-value	Odd ratio
Dyspnea stage				
Stage I	00 (0%)	2 (1,85%)		
Stage II	4 (7,41%)	6 (5,56%)		
Stage III	**23 (42,59%)**	**75 (69,44%)**	**0,001**	**2,8**
Stage IV	**27 (50%)**	**25 (23,15%)**		
PAS (mm Hg)				
0 à 90	**30 (55,56%)**	**16 (14,81%)**	**0,000**	**6,60**
91 à 139	21 (38,89%)	74 (68,52%)		1
140 and more	3 (5,56%)	18 (16,67%)	0,48	0,58
PAD (mm Hg)				
0 à 59	**18 (33,33%)**	**4 (3,70%)**	**0,000**	**10,4**
60 à 89	34 (62,96%)	79 (73,15%)		1
90 and over	2 (3,70%)	25(23,15%)	0,027	0,18

2.5.3 Bivariate analysis of biological factors

➢ **Distribution of patients by blood glucose level**

Table XII: Distribution by blood glucose level

Blood glucose (mmol/L)	Cases (%)	Witnesses (%)	OR	p	IC
Hypoglycemia	5 (9,26%)	1 (0,93%)	**11,7**	**0,027**	1,32 - 103,63
Normal blood glucose	38 (70,37%)	89 (82,41%)	1		
Hyperglycemia	11 (20,37%)	18 (16,67%)	1,43	0,43	0,61 - 3,31
Total	54 (100%)	108 (100%)			

In a univariate analysis, hypoglycemia was associated with mortality (p=0.021 and OR= 11.7). The mean blood glucose level in the study population was 5.68 ± 0.14 mmol/L. It was 5.75 ± 0.3 mmol/L in cases and 5.65

± 0.13 mmol/L in controls.

➢ **Distribution of patients by creatinine level**

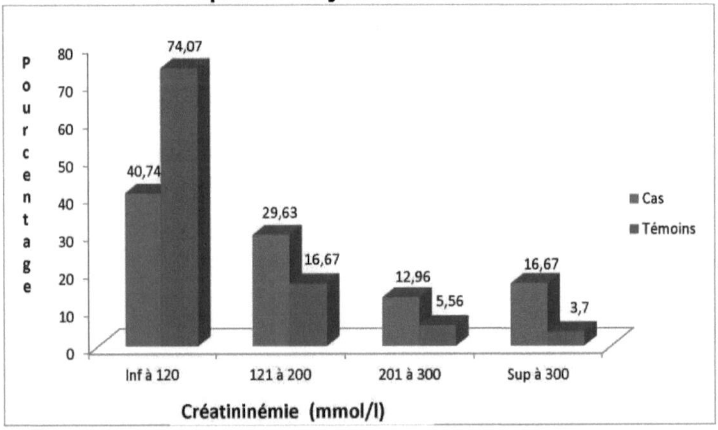

Figure 6: Distribution by creatinine level

Over half the cases had impaired renal function, and over half the controls had normal renal function. In univariate analysis, renal function impairment was associated with

mortality (p= 0.000). Mortality increased with increasing

creatinine (OR= 8 if creatinine above 300µmol/L).

The mean creatinine level of all patients was **141.5 ± 9.3µmol /L**. It was **195.8 ± 22.5µmol /L** for cases and **114, ± 6.9µmol /L** for controls.

- **Distribution of patients by glomerular filtration rate (GFR)**

Table XIII: GFR distribution (according to CKD-EPI)

GFR (ml/min	Case	Witnesses	OR	IC
Sup à 90	10 (18,52%)	38 (35,19%)	1	
90 à 60	11 (20, 37%)	37 (34,26%)	1,2	0,42 - 2,97
59 à 30	18 (33,33%)	25 (23,15%)	**2,73**	1,08 - 6,88
15 à 29	9 (16,67%)	7 (6,48%)	**4,58**	1,45 -16,36
0 à 14	6 (11,11%)	1 (0,93%)	**22,8**	2,45 - 211,75

p=0,001

Analysis of this table shows that decreasing glomerular filtration rate (GFR) was strongly associated with mortality (p= 0.001). Mortality increased with decreasing glomerular filtration rate (**OR= 22.8 for GFRs of 0 to 14 ml/min**).

The overall mean GFR for all patients was **70.8 ± 2.7ml/min**. It was **56 ± 4.7ml/min** for cases and **78.2 ± 3.1ml/min** for controls.

- **Distribution of patients by hemoglobin level**

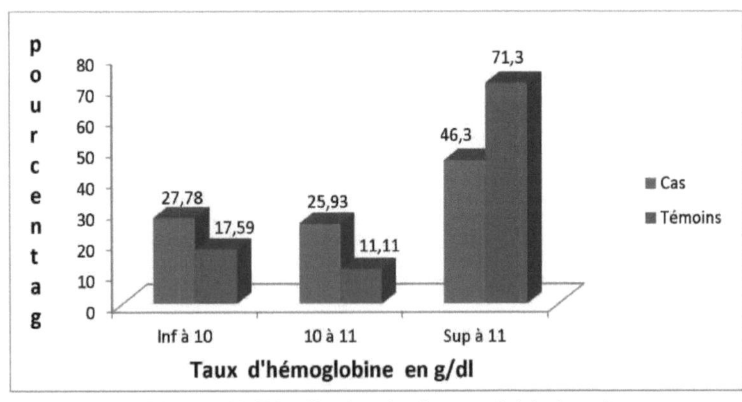

Figure 7: Distribution by hemoglobin level

In bivariate analysis, anemia was associated with mortality ($p= 0.006$).

The mean hemoglobin level in our study population was 11.6 ± 0.2 g/dl. It was 11.9 ± 0.2 g/dl for living patients and 10 ± 0.3 g/dl for deceased patients.

➢ **Distribution of patients according to natraemia**

Table XIV: Distribution according to natraemia

Natraemia	Case	Witnesses	OR	IC
Hyponatremia	**35 (64,81%)**	**27 (25%)**	**5,25**	**2,55 - 10,79**
Normal natraemia	18 (33,33%)	73 (67,59%)	1	
Hypernatremia	1 (1,85%)	8 (7,41%)	0,50	0,14 - 0,41

p= 0,000

This table shows that more than half the cases (64.81%) had hyponatremia and more than half the controls (67.59%) had normal natremia. Univariate analysis showed that hyponatremia was strongly associated with mortality (p= 0.000 and OR= 5.25).

The mean natraemia of all patients was **134.5 ± 0.6mmol/L**. It was **129 ± 1mmol/L** for cases and **137 ± 0.5mmol/L** for controls.

- **Summary of biological factors associated with mortality**

Table XV: Summary table of biological elements associated with mortality

Independent variable	Cases (%)	Controls (%)	p-value	Odd ratio
Blood glucose (mmol/L)				
Hypoglycemia	5 (9,26%)	1 (0,93%)	0,027	11,7
Normal blood glucose	38 (70,37%)	89 (82,41%)		
Hyperglycemia	11 (20,37%)	18 (16,67%)	0,43	
GFR (ml/min)				
Sup à 90	10 (18,52%)	38 (35,19%)		
90 à 60	11 (20, 37%)	37 (34,26%)		
59 à 30	18 (33,33%)	25 (23,15%)	0,033	2,73
15 à 29	9 (16,67%)	7 (6,48%)	0,010	4,88
0 à 14	6 (11,11%)	1 (0,93%)	0,001	22,8
Natremia (mmol/L)				
Hyponatremia	35 (64,81%)	27 (25%)	0,000	5,25
Normal natraemia	18 (33,33%)	73 (67,59%)		
Hypernatremia	1 (1,85%)	8 (7,41%)		
Hb level (g/dl)				
0 à 10	15 (27,78%)	19 (17,59%)		
10 à 11	14 (25,93%)	12 (11,11%)	0,005	3,59
Sup à 11	25 (46,30%)	77 (71,30%)		

2.5.4 Bivariate analysis of electrocardiographic factors

➢ **Distribution of patients according to conduction disorders**

Table XVI: Distribution by TDC

Conduction disorder	Cases (%)	Controls (%)	p	OR	IC
No	36 (66,67%)	91 (84,26%)	1		
Yes	**18 (33,33%)**	**17 (15,74%)**	**0,012**	**2,6**	**1,24 - 5,76**
Total	54 (100%)	108 (100%)			

Conduction disorder was associated with mortality (p= 0.012 and OR= 2.6).

2.5.5 Bivariate analysis of echocardiographic factors

➢ **Distribution of patients by LV end-diastolic diameter (LVEDD)**

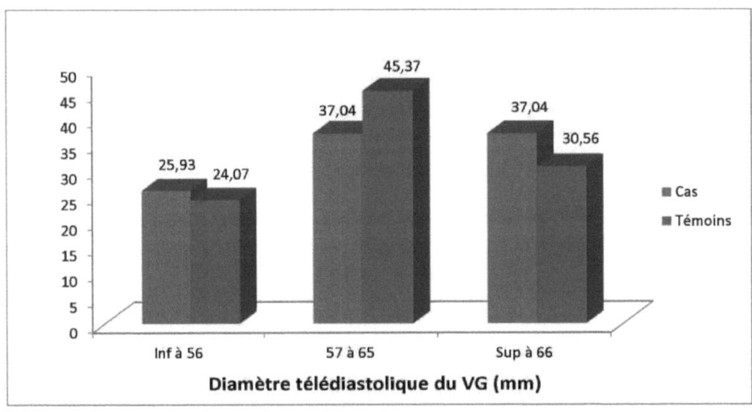

Figure 8: Distribution by left ventricular end-diastolic diameter.

According to the analysis, left ventricular dilatation was not associated with mortality (p= 0.57).

The mean DTDVG of the study population was **61.7 ± 0.7mm.** It was **62.4± 1.5mm** for cases and **61.3± 0.7mm** for controls.

➢ **Distribution of patients by left ventricular ejection fraction (LVEF)**

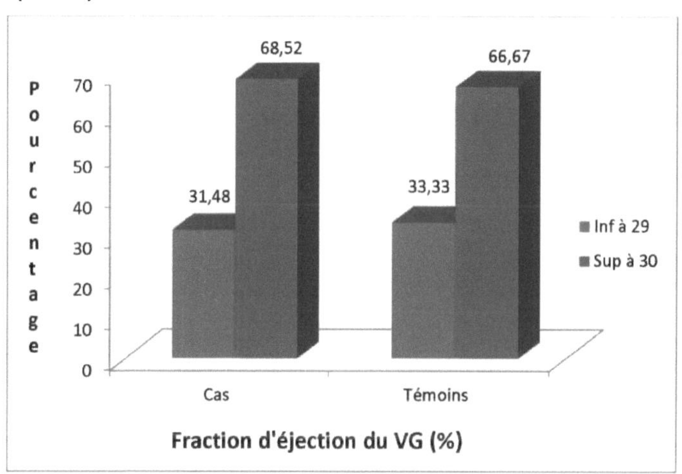

Figure 9: LVEF distribution

The figure above shows that impaired left ventricular ejection fraction was not associated with mortality (p= 0.81).

The mean LVEF of the study population was **33 ± 0.4%**. It was **34 ± 1.3%** in cases and **33 ± 0.8%** in controls.

- **Distribution of patients according to filling pressures left ventricle (E/A).**

Table XVII: Distribution by filling pressure (E/A).

E/A	Cases (%)	Controls (%)	p	OR	IC
Less than 2	13 (24,07%)	45 (41,67%)	1		
Sup à 2	41 (75,93%)	63 (58,33%)	0,03	2,25	1,08 - 4,68
Total	54 (100%)	108 (100%)			

The table above shows that 76% of cases and 58% of controls had elevated filling pressures. The analysis noted that elevated filling pressures were associated with mortality (p= 0.03).

- **TAPSE (Tricuspid Annular Posterior Systolic Excursion) distribution**

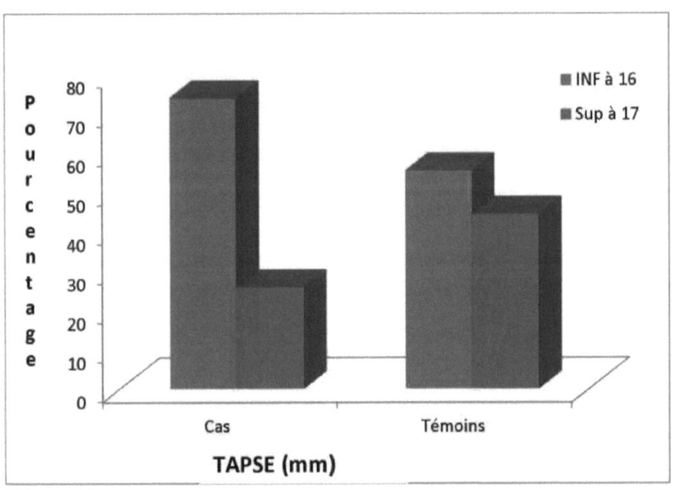

Figure 10: Distribution by TAPSE

According to the figure above, 74% of cases and 55% of controls had impaired TAPSE.

The mean TAPSE in our study population was **15.1 ± 0.3 mm**. It was **13.9 ± 0.6** mm in deceased patients and **15.7 ± 0.3** mm in living patients. The analysis concluded that impaired right ventricular systolic function (RVSSF) was associated with mortality (p= 0.02).

- **Distribution of patients by systolic pulmonary arterial pressure (SPAP)**

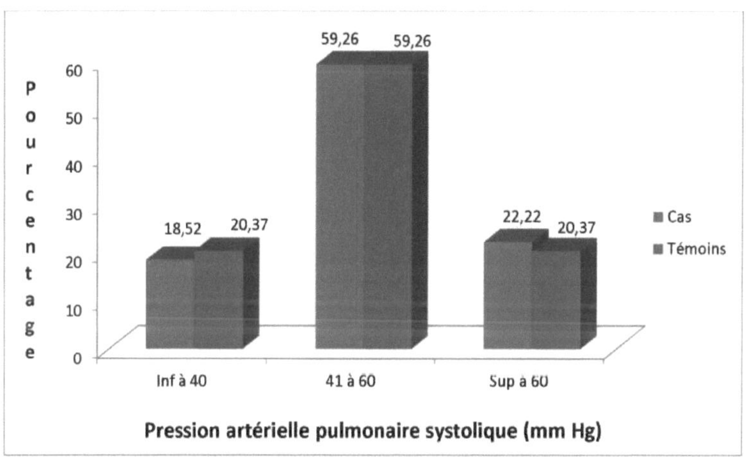

Figure 11: Breakdown by PAPS

Sixty percent of cases and controls had PAPS between 41 and 60 mm Hg. Analysis showed that pulmonary hypertension was not associated with mortality (p= 0.9).

The mean PAPS of the study population was **51.6 ± 1 mm Hg**. It was 52.5 ± 1.8 mm Hg for cases and 51.2 ± 1.3 mm Hg for controls.

➢ **Summary of echocardiographic factors associated with mortality**

Table XVIII: Summary table of echocardiographic features associated with mortality

Independent variable	Cases (%)	Controls (%)	p-value	Odd ratio
E/A				
Less than 2	13 (24,07%)	45 (41,67%)		
Sup à 2	**41 (75,93%)**	**63 (58,33%)**	**0,03**	**2,25**
TAPSE (mm)				
under 16	**40 (74,07%)**	**60 (55,56%)**	**0,02**	**2,28**
Sup à 17	14 (25,93%)	48 (44,44%)		

2.5.4 Bivariate analysis of therapeutic factors

➢ **Distribution of patients according to beta-blocker treatment**

Table XIX: Distribution according to beta-blocker treatment

Beta-blocker treatment	Case	Witnesses
No	48 (88,89%)	88 (81,48%)
Yes	6 (11,11%)	20 (18,52%)
Total	54 (100%)	108 (100%)

P=0,22

Beta-blockers were prescribed less frequently in both cases and controls. The analysis shows that treatment with beta-blockers was not associated with mortality (p= 0.22).

- **Distribution of patients according to spironolactone treatment**

Table XX: Distribution according to spironolactone treatment

Spironolactone treatment	Case	Witnesses
No	33 (61,11%)	18 (16,67%)
Yes	21 (38,89%)	90 (83,33%)
Total	54 (100%)	108 (100%)

Prescription of spironolactone was beneficial for survival in patients with heart failure (OR= -12)

- **Distribution of patients according to tonicardiac treatment**

Table XXI: Distribution according to tonicardiac treatment

Treatment with tonicardiacs	Case	Witnesses
No	31 (57,41%)	11 (10,19%)
Yes	23 (42,59)	97 (89,81%)
Total	54 (100%)	108 (100%)

P= 0,000

Tonicardiac use was associated with mortality (p= 0.000 OR 5.5).

2.5.7 Multivariate analysis of factors associated with mortality

Table XXII: Multivariate analysis of factors associated with mortality

Variables	Hospital mortality			
	OR	p-value	[IC].	
ATCD IC				
No	1			
Yes	1,38	0,502	0,53	3,58
Stage of dyspnea				
Stage I	1			
Stage II	0,96	0,91	0,16	5,48
Stage III	**2,7**	**0,005**	**0,10**	**0,66**
Stage IV	1			
NOT				
0 to 90 mm Hg	**4,38**	**0,003**	**1,62**	**11,82**
90 to 139 mm Hg	1			
Above 140 mm Hg	0,74	0,709	0,15	3,58
Creatinine clearance				
0 to 14 ml/min	2,74	0,438	0,21	35,26
15 to 29 ml/min	2,59	0,222	0,56	11,96
30 to 59 ml/min	2,27	0,145	0,75	6,83
60 to 90 ml/min	1,01	0,980	0,32	3,21
90 to more	1			
Natraemia				
Hyponatremia	**2,95**	**0,017**	**1,21**	**7,21**
Normal natraemia	1			
hypernatremia	1,24	0,857	1,14	12,10
Hemoglobin level				
Below 10 g/dl	2,19	0,139	0,77	12,10
10 to 11 g/dl	**3,77**	**0,029**	**1,14**	**12,10**
11 to more	1			

In multivariate analysis by stepwise regression, the factors that were associated with mortality in systolic heart failure were:

- ✓ stage III dyspnea with a p-value of 0.005, an OR of 2.7 and [CI] 0.10 - 0.66 ;
- ✓ PAS less than 90 mm Hg with a p-value of 0.003, an OR of 4.38 and [CI] 1.62 - 11.82 ;
- ✓ hyponatremia with a p-value of 0.017, an OR of 2.95 and [CI] 1.21 - 7.21.
- ✓ anemia with p-value 0.029, OR 3.77 and [CI] 1.14 - 12.10

The model specification has been verified using the Roc statistical method.

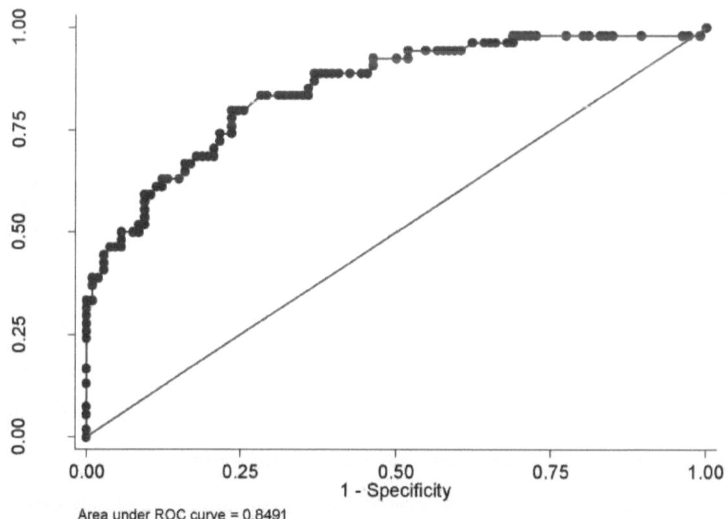

Figure 12: Sensitivity and specificity of factors associated with mortality according to the Roc curve.

The area under the curve was 0.85, i.e. within the range [0.8 - 0.9], which means that the specificity and sensitivity of these factors associated with mortality were excellent.

2.5.8 Proposal of a score predictive of in-hospital mortality in systolic heart failure

The score model: the items

1- Stage III dyspnea: p= 0.005
2- Arterial hypotension (PAS less than 90 mm Hg): p= 0.003
3- History of heart failure: p= 0.502
4- Hyponatremia: p= 0.017
5- anemia: 0.029

Criteria :

- **P< 0.01 strong association = 3 points**
- **P= 0.01 to 0.05 weak association = 2 points**
- **P> 0.05 no association = 1 point**

2.6 DISCUSSION

2.6.1 The limits of our study

The limitations of our study were, firstly, incomplete clinical records. Secondly, as our data collection was based on retrospective data, we were unable to prove the links between all the factors associated with mortality in systolic heart failure described in the literature, as would have been the case with cohort or prospective case-control studies. And finally, we only assessed factors associated with in-hospital mortality; and this cannot be extrapolated to predict mortality in patients discharged alive and followed as outpatients.

Despite our limitations, we were able to identify factors associated with mortality in systolic heart failure, which we will compare with other studies and with data in the literature.

2.6.2 Socio-demographic factors

a- age and gender

The mean age of the study population was : 58.24 ± 1.4 years. The mean age of cases was 57.38 ± 2.3 years and that of controls 58.66 ± 1.7 years. Our results were similar to those of Bivigou et al in Gabon, who found 55.8 years for the study population, 55 years for deceased patients and 57.4 years for living patients [49], Pio et al in Togo, who found 57. 4 years for deceased patients [5], and Kheyi et al in Morocco, who found 60.9 years [50].

However, these African data differed from those for Europe, with an average age of 75 years for patients who died and 67 years for those who lived in Poland [51], and 86.4 years for those who died in France [52]. This difference between developed countries and Africa could be explained by a delay in diagnosis and a difficulty in providing adequate care due to poverty.

The majority of our study population was male, with a sex ratio of 1.7 in cases and 1.4 in controls. This has been found in several studies [49-51].

These results were in line with the literature, which classifies male sex as a poor prognostic factor in heart failure [53,54].

2.6.3 Factors associated with mortality

- **Socio-demographic factors**

a- age of heart failure

The mean overall duration of heart failure was 13.6 ± 1.6 months. The mean duration for **cases was 21.3 ± 3.2** months. It was **9.7 ± 1.3** months for controls. Mohamed et al in Algeria made the same observation [4]. This is in line with the literature, which considers heart failure to be a chronic pathology in most cases.

In bivariate analysis, the age of heart failure was associated with mortality (p=0.003 and OR= 4.25 from 13 months).

b- hospital stay

The mean length of hospital stay for our study population was 10.2 ± 0.5 days. Patients who died had an average stay of 11.5 ± 1.2 days. Controls had an average stay of 9.6 ± 0.5 days. Our result was close to some African studies. The mean stay for deceased patients was 12, 15 and 17 days respectively in Morocco [50], Gabon [49] and Congo [55].

➢ **Clinical factors**

a- Stages of dyspnea

Almost all patients who died (92.59%) were admitted with NYHA stage III and IV dyspnea. More than half (70%) of living patients were admitted with NYHA stage III dyspnea. In multivariate analysis, NYHA stage III dyspnea was strongly associated with mortality (p-value 0.007, OR 2.7).

Our results were similar to those of numerous studies, notably Keita et al in Guinea Conakry, who found 92% of patients in stages III and IV [56], Kingue et al in Cameroon found 53% of patients in stages III and IV, Kheyi et al in Morocco found 54% of patients in stages III and IV [50], Mohamed et al in Algeria found 57% of patients in stages III and IV, and Abraham et al in the USA found 44% of stage IV dyspnea in deceased patients [57].

Stages III and IV, widely found in our regions, reflect the late diagnosis and severity of heart failure. This could be explained by poverty and ignorance, limiting access to care for the most disadvantaged populations.

The disparity in results between different studies is explained by the subjective nature of dyspnoea. Dyspnoea stage is a prognostic criterion often used, but unfortunately it is widely criticized for its subjective nature [58, 59]. However, it remains the benchmark for categorizing patients and determining therapeutic indications.

b- Blood pressure

The mean systolic blood pressure in our study population was 106.6 ± 2.1 mm Hg. It was 80 ± 4 mm Hg in deceased patients, and 115.4 ± 1.8 mm Hg in living patients. In both bivariate and multivariate analyses, the drop in SBP was strongly associated with mortality (p= 0.003, OR 4.38 in multivariate analysis).

The mean diastolic blood pressure of all patients was 69 **±** 1.6 mm Hg. It was 54.4± 3.2 mm Hg in deceased patients and 76.4± 1.3 mm Hg in living patients. In bivariate analysis, PAD was associated with mortality (p=0.000 and OR= 10.4).

A number of studies have shown that arterial hypotension is a poor prognostic factor in heart failure. Hypotension increased the risk of death by a factor of eight (08) in a Gabonese series [49], and by a factor of four (04) in a series from Uganda [60] and Algeria [4].

These results are in line with the literature, which considers hypotension to be a poor prognostic factor, especially when associated with a sign of low output, thus contraindicating the drug classes that are essential in the treatment of heart failure [61,62].

c- Heart rate

The mean heart rate in our study population was 99.8 ± 2 bpm. It was 100.2 ± 3.5 bpm in deceased patients and 99.7± 2 bpm in living patients. In our analysis, high heart rate was not associated with mortality.

Our result contrasts with the literature, which considers a rapid heart rate to be a poor prognostic factor [25, 63, 64].

But from a pathophysiological point of view, rapid heart rate is one of the compensatory signs involved in heart failure. It would therefore be critical to consider it as a prognostic factor.

- **Biological factors**

a- Creatinine levels and glomerular filtration rate

The mean creatinine level of all patients was 141.5 ± 9.3 µmol /L. It was 195.8± 22.5 µmol/L in deceased patients and 114.3 ± 7 µmol/L in living patients.

The overall mean glomerular filtration rate (GFR) for all patients was 70.8 ± 2.7 ml/min. It was 56 ± 4.7 ml/min in deceased patients and 78.2 ± 3 ml/min in living patients.

Renal failure was strongly associated with mortality in our study. Most studies have also made the same finding. In Gabon, 56.4% of patients who died had renal insufficiency [49], while in Cameroon, 20% of patients with heart failure had renal insufficiency [6]. Polish studies found that increased serum creatinine was predictive of in-hospital death in patients hospitalized for heart failure [51, 65].

The results of our study are in line with the literature, which affirms that the existence of renal failure leads to excess morbidity and mortality, especially in the elderly, due to hydro-electrolytic disorders and disturbances in blood pressure [66].

Half (55%) of patients with chronic heart failure, especially advanced heart failure, have reduced renal function [67]. This considerably worsens the prognosis of heart failure. Mortality increases proportionally with the fall in glomerular filtration rate [68].

Renal failure, an independent factor in heart failure mortality, is multifactorial. It may be an early complication of hypertension in black subjects [69], and may then be associated with heart failure. It may also be the consequence of low renal output in heart failure with impaired LVEF.

b- Hemoglobin level

The mean hemoglobin level in our study population was 11.6 ± 0.2 g/dl. It was 11.9 ± 0.2 g/dl for living patients and 10 ± 0.3 g/dl for deceased patients. In both bivariate and multivariate analyses, anemia was associated with mortality (p= 0.029 and OR= 3.77 in multivariate analysis).

The result of our study is similar to that of Bivigou et al in Gabon, who found a mean hemoglobin level in the study population of 10.7 ± 2 g/dl, 9.9 ± 2.4 g/dl in deceased patients and 11.1 ± 1.7 g/dl in living patients [49]. In Morocco, Kheyi et al reported that 21% of heart failure patients had anaemia [50] and in Uganda, Okello et al reported 18.3% [60].

The existence of anemia is a severe prognostic factor [70], although the interaction between anemia and heart failure is not yet fully understood, and it is still difficult to say which of the two is responsible for the other's poor prognosis [71].

Anemia leads to a reduction in functional capacity for exercise and is often considered an independent factor in mortality [48].

c- Natremia

The mean natraemia in our study population was 134.5 ± 0.6 mmol/L. It was 129 ± 1 mmol/L in deceased patients and 137 ± 0.5 mmol/L in living patients.

In both bivariate and multivariate analyses, hyponatremia was strongly associated with mortality (p-value 0.017, OR 2.95 in multivariate analysis). Other studies have confirmed that hyponatremia is associated with an increased risk of mortality, particularly in the elderly [64,72].

Among biological prognostic factors, studies have confirmed the major contribution of BNP in the prognostic evaluation and risk stratification of patients with systolic heart failure, irrespective of LVEF level. Increased BNP levels are associated with mortality [73, 74].

- **Electrocardiographic and echocardiographic factors Doppler**

a- Conduction disorders

In our study, conduction disorder was associated with mortality (p= 0.012 and OR= 2.6).

Complete left bundle branch block was not associated with mortality in heart failure.

The same finding was made in a Gabonese study, which showed that isolated complete left bundle-branch block was not associated with mortality. On the other hand, the association of complete branch block and severely impaired LVEF increased the risk of mortality [49].

b- Left ventricular ejection fraction (LVEF)

The mean LVEF in our study population was 33 ± 0.4%. It was 34 ± 1.3% in deceased patients and 33 ± 0.8% in living patients. Our analysis showed that impaired left ventricular ejection fraction was not associated with mortality (p= 0.81).

Numerous African studies have reported that impaired LVEF is associated with mortality [48 ,49 ,60 ,75].

Furthermore, some studies have found no link between LVEF impairment and mortality in heart failure [51, 76]. Other studies conclude that the prognostic value of LVEF disappears below 30% [77, 78].

This disparity in results between studies could be explained by the fact that echocardiographic assessment of LVEF is less reliable than other techniques, notably angiography or isotopic LVEF.

Other parameters such as restrictive and irreversible mitral profile and ventricular asynchronism have a negative prognostic value.

c- Left ventricular end-diastolic diameter (LVEDD)

The mean DTDVG in our study population was 61.7 ± 0.7 mm. It was 62.4 ± 1.5 mm in deceased patients and 61.3 ± 0.7 mm in living patients. According to our analysis, left ventricular dilatation was not associated with mortality (p= 0.57).

Our result is similar to that of Bivigou et al, who found a mean DTDVG of 62.5 ± 8.7 mm in deceased patients and 59.18 ± 9.6 mm in living patients [49].

d- Systolic pulmonary arterial pressure (SPAP)

The mean PAPS in the study population was 51.6 ± ImmHg. It was 52.5 ± 1.8 mmHg in deceased patients and 51.2 ± 1.3 mmHg in living patients.

Analysis showed that pulmonary hypertension was not associated with mortality (p= 0.9).

Our results are in line with those of Bivigou et al, who found that elevated PAPS was not associated with mortality [49].

On the other hand, Abramson et al found a link between elevated PAPS and mortality [79].

e- La TAPSE

The mean TAPSE in our study population was 15.1 ± 0.3 mm. It was 13.9 ± 0.6 mm in deceased patients and 15.7 ± 0.3 mm in living patients. The analysis concluded that impaired right ventricular systolic function (RVSSF) was associated with mortality (p= 0.02).

Some studies have concluded that the assessment of right ventricular systolic function is of greater prognostic value than PAPS [80, 81]. This is because impairment of right ventricular systolic function is the ultimate outcome of left ventricular damage. Moreover, as the right ventricle is the preload for the left ventricle, its damage will lead to low flow, which will be highly deleterious for organ perfusion, with multi-visceral damage (brain, kidneys, heart, liver, etc.), resulting in a high risk of death.

- **Therapeutic factors**

Prescription of spironolactone was beneficial for survival in patients with heart failure (OR= -12)

The use of tonicardiacs was associated with mortality (p= 0.000 OR 5.5). It should be noted that this association was not directly linked to the prescription of tonicardiacs, but to the state of shock for which tonicardiacs were widely prescribed. Alakoua et al in Burkina Faso reported 48% of deaths in patients on dobutamine [83]. Shock results in visceral hypoperfusion, which is responsible for death.

- **Multivariate analysis of factors associated with mortality**

In multivariate stepwise regression analysis, the factors associated with mortality in systolic heart failure were: dyspnea stage III, PAS below 90 mm Hg, hyponatremia and anemia.

In view of the factors associated with mortality in systolic heart failure, verified by statistical regression and with excellent specificity and sensitivity according to the roc curve (area under the curve equal to 0.85), we propose a score predictive of intra-hospital mortality in systolic heart failure.

Proposal of a score predictive of in-hospital mortality in systolic heart failure

Table XXIII: Predictive mortality score model

Items	p-value	Points
Hypotension (PAS below 90 mm Hg)	0,003	**3**
NYHA stage III	0,005	**3**
Hyponatremia	0,017	**2**
Anemia	0,029	**2**
History of heart failure	0,502	**1**
Total		**11 points**

The combination of these factors would have a negative prognostic value in systolic heart failure.

It would be desirable to initiate a multicenter cohort study to validate this score and stratify it into low, moderate and high risk, each of which needs to be statistically verified.

CONCLUSION

Given that heart failure is a chronic pathology, despite diagnostic and therapeutic advances in its management, it constitutes a public health problem due to its high morbidity and mortality, especially in countries with limited resources. The results of our study show that the factors associated with high mortality are sociodemographic (antecedent CI, duration of CI evolution), clinical (arterial hypotension, stage III dyspnea) and paraclinical (renal failure, hyponatremia and anemia). It is important to stratify the risk of mortality associated with systolic heart failure, once the negative prognostic factors have been identified. This stratification will help optimize the management of heart failure.

It is therefore necessary to initiate multicenter cohort studies to stratify the risk of mortality in systolic heart failure in a context of limited resources.

SUGGESTIONS

At the end of our study, we offer suggestions for improving the prognosis of hospitalized heart failure patients.

To the Minister of Public Health

- ✓ Combating cardiovascular risk factors through primary prevention.
- ✓ Making emergency medicines available and accessible
- ✓ cardiovascular,
- ✓ Making BNP assays available to hospitals in
- ✓ reference,
- ✓ Subsidize cardiovascular drugs,
- ✓ **To the Head of Cardiology**
- ✓ Initiate a cohort study on the prognosis of heart failure to better identify prognostic factors,
- ✓ Set up an inpatient heart failure registry.

REFERENCES

1. Hebbar E. Comparison of prognostic factors for systolic heart failure: impact of heart disease etiology. University of Lillle2; 2014.
2. Stewart S, MacIntyre K, Hole DJ, Capewell S, McMurray JJV. More 'malignant' than cancer? Five-year survival following a first admission for heart failure. European Journal of Heart Failure. 2001; 3: 315-22.
3. Ponikowski P, Voors AA, Anker SD, Bueno H, Cleland JGF, Coats AJS, et al. 2016 ESC Guidelines for the diagnosis and treatment of acute and chronic heart failure. European Heart Journal. 2016;37: 2129-200.
4. Mohammed HA. Analysis of predictors of short- and medium-term mortality in chronic systolic heart failure. Oran 1 University; 2015.
5. Pio M, Afassinou Y, Pessinaba S, Baragou S, N'djao J, Atta B, et al. Epidemiology and etiologies of heart failure in Lomé. The Pan African Medical Journal. 2014;18.
6. Kingue S, Dzudie A, Menanga A, Akono M, Ouankou M, Muna W. A new look at adult chronic heart failure in Africa in the era of Doppler echocardiography: experience from the medicine department of Yaoundé General Hospital. Annales de Cardiologie et d'Angéiologie.2005;54:276-83.
7. Adjougoulta A. Epidemiological, clinical and evolutionary aspects of heart failure at the National Reference General Hospital of N'Djamena. University of N'Djamena; 2012.
8. Ouedraogo M. Heart failure: epidemiological, clinical, paraclinical, therapeutic and evolutionary aspects. A propos de 207 cas colligés au CHUYO. Joseph Ki Zerbo University; 2014.
9. Temoua N. Heart failure: epidemiological, clinical and evolutionary aspects. A propos de 172 cas colligés dans le service de cardiologie du CHU Yalgado Ouedraogo. Université Joseph Ki Zerbo; 2006.
10. Juillière YBJ al. Cardiology and vascular diseases. In: Masson. France; 2007. p. 663-72.

11. Cohen A. The fundamentals of cardiovascular pathology. In: Les fondamentaux de la pathologie cardiovasculaire: Enseignement intégré-sytème cardiovasculaire. Masson. France; 2014. p. 111-45.
12. Writing committee members, Hunt SA, Abraham WT, Chin MH, Feldman AM, Francis GS, et al. ACC/AHA 2005 Guideline Update for the Diagnosis and Management of Chronic Heart Failure in the Adult: A Report of the American College of Cardiology/American Heart Association Task Force on Practice Guidelines (Writing Committee to Update the 2001 Guidelines for the Evaluation and Management of Heart Failure): Developed in Collaboration With the American College of Chest Physicians and the International Society for Heart and Lung Transplantation: Endorsed by the Heart Rhythm Society. Circulation. 2005;112(12).
13. Goodlin SJ, Hauptman PJ, Arnold R, Grady K, Hershberger RE, Kutner J, et al. Consensus statement: Palliative and supportive care in advanced heart failure. Journal of Cardiac Failure. 2004; 10: 200-9.
14. Haute autorité de santé. Heart failure. 2014.
15. Ho KK, Pinsky JL, Kannel WB, Levy D. The epidemiology of heart failure: the Framingham Study. J Am Coll Cardiol.1993; 22: 6A-13A.
16. Cowie M. Hospitalization of patients with heart failure. A population-based study. European Heart Journal. 2002; 23: 877-85.
17. Connolly S. Meta-analysis of the implantable cardioverter defibrillator secondary prevention trials. European Heart Journal. 2000; 21: 2071-8.
18. Redfield MM, Rodeheffer RJ, Jacobsen SJ, Mahoney DW, Bailey KR, Burnett JC. Plasma brain natriuretic peptide concentration: impact of age and gender. Am J Cardiol. 2002; 40: 976-82.
19. Keta A. Heart failure Geneva. 2017.
20. Mosterd A, Hoes AW. Clinical epidemiology of heart failure. Heart. 2007; 93:1137-46.
21. Hunt SA, Abraham WT, Chin MH, Feldman AM, Francis GS, Ganiats TG,

et al. 2009 focused update incorporated into the ACC/AHA 2005 Guidelines for the Diagnosis and Management of Heart Failure in Adults: Circulation. 2009; 119: 391- 479.

22. Lloyd-Jones D, Adams R, Carnethon M, De Simone G, Ferguson TB, Flegal K, et al. Heart disease and stroke statistics--2009 update: a report from the American Heart Association Statistics Committee and Stroke Statistics Subcommittee. Circulation. 2009; 119:480–6.

23. Lee DS, Austin PC, Rouleau JL, Liu PP, Naimark D, Tu JV. Predicting mortality among patients hospitalized for heart failure: derivation and validation of a clinical model. JAMA. 2003; 290: 2581 –7.

24. Bourassa MG, Gurné O, Bangdiwala SI, Ghali JK, Young JB, Rousseau M, et al. Natural history and patterns of current practice in heart failure. The Studies of Left Ventricular Dysfunction (SOLVD) Investigators. Am J Cardiol. 1993; 22: 14A- 19A.

25. Tribouilloy C, Rusinaru D, Mahjoub H, Tartiere J-M, Kesri-Tartiere L, Godard S, et al. Prognostic impact of diabetes mellitus in patients with heart failure and preserved ejection fraction: a prospective five-year study.Heart. 2008; 94:1450–5.

26. MacIntyre K., Capewell S., Stewart S., Chalmers J.W.T., Boyd J., Finlayson A., et al. Evidence of Improving Prognosis in Heart Failure. Circulation.2000; 102: 1126–31.

27. Likoff MJ, Chandler SL, Kay HR. Clinical determinants of mortality in chronic congestive heart failure secondary to idiopathic dilated or to ischemic cardiomyopathy. Am J Cardiol.1987; 59: 634–8.

28. Goldberg RJ, Ciampa J, Lessard D, Meyer TE, Spencer FA. Long-term survival after heart failure: a contemporary population-based perspective. Arch Intern Med. 2007; 167: 490–6.

29. The Seattle Heart Failure Model: prediction of survival in heart failure. - PubMed - NCBI. 2019.

30. Hillege HL, Girbes AR, de Kam PJ, Boomsma F, de Zeeuw D,

Charlesworth A, et al. Renal function, neurohormonal activation, and survival in patients with chronic heart failure. Circulation. 2000; 102: 203-10.

31. Gomes JA, Mehta D, Ip J, Winters SL, Camunas J, Ergin A, et al. Predictors of long-term survival in patients with malignant ventricular arrhythmias. Am J Cardiol.1997; 79: 1054-60.

32. Stein GY, Kremer A, Shochat T, Bental T, Korenfeld R, Abramson E, et al. The diversity of heart failure in a hospitalized population: the role of age. J Card Fail. 2012; 18: 645-53.

33. Nagueh SF, Smiseth OA, Appleton CP, Byrd BF, Dokainish H, Edvardsen T, et al. Recommendations for the Evaluation of Left Ventricular Diastolic Function by Echocardiography: An Update from the American Society of Echocardiography and the European Association of Cardiovascular Imaging. Journal of the American Society of Echocardiography. 2016; 29: 277-314.

34. The Consensus Trial Study Group*. Effects of Enalapril on Mortality in Severe Congestive Heart Failure. New England Journal of Medicine. 1987; 316: 1429-35.

35. Garg R, Yusuf S. Overview of randomized trials of angiotensin-converting enzyme inhibitors on mortality and morbidity in patients with heart failure. Collaborative Group on ACE Inhibitor Trials. JAMA.1995; 273: 1450-6.

36. Granger CB, McMurray JJ, Yusuf S, Held P, Michelson EL, Olofsson B, et al. Effects of candesartan in patients with chronic heart failure and reduced left-ventricular systolic function intolerant to angiotensin-converting-enzyme inhibitors: the CHARM-Alternative trial.

37. The Cardiac Insufficiency Bisoprolol Study II (CIBIS-II): a randomised trial. The Lancet. 1999; 353: 9-13.

38. Effect of metoprolol CR/XL in chronic heart failure: Metoprolol CR/XL Randomised Intervention Trial in Congestive Heart Failure (MERIT-HF). Lancet.1999; 353: 2001-7.

39. Pitt B, Zannad F, Remme WJ, Cody R, Castaigne A, Perez A, et al. The Effect of Spironolactone on Morbidity and Mortality in Patients with Severe Heart Failure. New England Journal of Medicine. 1999; 341: 709-17.
40. Swedberg K, Komajda M, Bohm M, Borer JS, Ford I, Dubost-Brama A, et al. Ivabradine and outcomes in chronic heart failure (SHIFT): a randomised placebo- controlled study. The Lancet. 2010; 376: 875-85.
41. The Effect of Digoxin on Mortality and Morbidity in Patients with Heart Failure. New England Journal of Medicine.1997; 336: 525-33.
42. King JB, Bress AP, Reese AD, Munger MA. Neprilysin Inhibition in Heart Failure with Reduced Ejection Fraction: A Clinical Review. Pharmacotherapy: The Journal of Human Pharmacology and Drug Therapy. 2015; 35: 823-37.
43. Taylor AL, Ziesche S, Yancy C, Carson P, D'Agostino R, Ferdinand K, et al. Combination of Isosorbide Dinitrate and Hydralazine in Blacks with Heart Failure. New England Journal of Medicine. 2004; 351: 2049-57.
44. Abraham WT, Fisher WG, Smith AL, Delurgio DB, Leon AR, Loh E, et al. Cardiac Resynchronization in Chronic Heart Failure. New England Journal of Medicine. 2002; 346: 1845-53.
45. Cleland JGF, Daubert J-C, Erdmann E, Freemantle N, Gras D, Kappenberger L, et al. The Effect of Cardiac Resynchronization on Morbidity and Mortality in Heart Failure. New England Journal of Medicine. 2005; 352: 1539-49.
46. Hosenpud JD, Bennett LE, Keck BM, Boucek MM, Novick RJ. The Registry of the International Society for Heart and Lung Transplantation: seventeenth official report-2000. J Heart Lung Transplant. 2000; 19: 909-31.
47. Hung MJ, Cherng WJ, Kuo LT, Wang CH. Effect of verapamil in elderly patients with left ventricular diastolic dysfunction as a cause of congestive heart failure. Int J Clin Pract. 2002; 56: 57-62.

48. Makubi A, Hage C, Lwakatare J, Kisenge P, Makani J, Rydén L, et al. Contemporary aetiology, clinical characteristics and prognosis of adults with heart failure observed in a tertiary hospital in Tanzania: the prospective Tanzania Heart Failure (TaHeF) study. Heart. 2014; 100: 1235-41.
49. Bivigou EA, Allognon MC, Ndoume F, Mipinda JB, Nzengue EE. Lethality of heart failure at the Centre Hospitalier Universitaire de Libreville (CHUL) and associated factors. Pan African Medical Journal. 2018;31.
50. Kheyi J, Benelmakki A, Bouzelmat H, Chaib A. Epidemiology and management of heart failure in a Moroccan center. Pan African Medical Journal. 2016 ;24.
51. Ostrowska M, Ostrowski A, Luczak M, Jaguszewski M, Adamski P, Bellwon J, et al. Basic laboratory parameters as predictors of in-hospital death in patients with acute decompensated heart failure: data from a large single-centre cohort. Kardiologia Polska. 2016;157-63.
52. Amélie G. Mortality due to heart failure in France, evolutions 20002010. 386e ed. Nice 2014;21 -2.
53. JuillièreY, BerderV, Brembilla-Perrot B, Selton-Suty C. Response to drug treatments for heart failure according to gender. Arch Mal Coeur 2004;97: 1216-20.
54. Ghali JK, Krause-Steinrauf HJ, Adams KF, et al. Gender differences in advanced heart failure: insights from the BEST study. J Am Coll Cardiol 2003;42: 2128-34.
55. Ikama MS. Heart failure in the elderly in Brazaville: clinical, etiological and evolutionary aspects. 68e éd. 2008;257-60.
56. Keita M, Boitrin TI, Dombouya N, Touré BM,Agbo-Panzo D, Magassouba, DF, et al. Heart failure of hypertensive origin comparative multicenter study and prognosis from 73 cases in Conakry. Guinée Médicale 2002; 35:313.
57. Abraham WT, Fonarow GC, Albert NM, Stough WG, Gheorghiade M, Greenberg BH, et al. Predictors of In-Hospital Mortality in Patients

Hospitalized for Heart Failure. Journal of the American College of Cardiology. 2008; 52: 347-56.

58. Madsen BK, Hansen JF, Stockholm KH, et al. Chronic congestive heart failure. Description and survival of 190 consecutive patients with a diagnosis of chronic congestive heart failure based on clinical signs and symptoms. Eur Heart J 1994;15: 303-10.
59. Keogh AM, Baron DW, Hickie JB. Prognostic guides in patients with idiopathic or ischemic dilated cardiomyopathy assessed for cardiac transplantation. Am J Cardiol 1990;65: 903-8.
60. Okello S, Rogers O, Byamugisha A, Rwebembera J, Buda AJ. Characteristics of acute heart failure hospitalizations in a general medical ward in Southwestern Uganda. International Journal of Cardiology. 2014; 176: 1233-4.
61. Anguita M, Arizon JM, Bueno G, et al. Clinical and haemodynamic predictors of survival in patients aged < 65 years with severe congestive heart failure secondary to ischemic or nonischemic cardiomyopathy. Am J Cardiol 1993;72: 413-7.
62. Campana C, Gavazzi A, Berzuini C, et al. Predictors of prognosis in patients awaiting heart transplantation. J Heart Lung Transpl 1993;12: 756-65.
63. Nul DR, Doval HC, Grancelli HO, et al,GESICA-GEMA Investigators. Heart rate is a marker of amiodarone mortality reduction in severe heart failure. J Am Coll Cardiol 1997;29: 1199-205.
64. Aaronson KD, Schawartz JS, Chen TM, Wong KL, Goin JE, Mancini, DM. Development and prospective validation of a clinical index to predict survival in ambulatory patients referred for cardiac transplant evaluation. Circulation 1997;95: 2660-7.
65. Biegus J, Zymlinski R, Szachniewicz J et al. Clinical characteristics and predictors of in-hospital mortality in 270 consecutive patients hospitalized due to acute heart failure in a single cardiology center during one year. Kardiol Pol. 2011; 69(10): 997-1005.

66. Zannad F, Briançon S, Juillière Y, et al. Incidence, clinical and etiologic features, and outcomes of advanced chronic heart failure: the EPICAL study. J Am Coll Cardiol 1999; 33: 734-42.
67. McDonagh TA, Gardner RS, Clark AL,, Darcie HJ, eds. Oxford Textbook of Heart Failure Oxford , Oxford University Press, 2011 : 281 - 381.
68. Go AS, Chertow GM, Fand Mc Culloch CE, Hsu C. Chronic kidney disease and the riskes of death, cardiovascular events and hospitalization . N Engl J Med 2004 ; 351 : 1296 - 3051 7.
69. Amah G, Lévy B I. Particularities of hypertension in black-African subjects. STV. 2007; 19(10): 519-525.
70. Ezekowitz JA, McAlister FA, Armstrong PW. Anemia is common in heart failure and is associated with poor outcomes. Insights from a cohort of 12065 patients with new-onset heart failure. Circulation 2003;107: 223-5.
71. Kalra PR, Collier T, Cowie MR, et al. Haemoglobin concentration and prognosis in new cases of heart failure. Lancet 2003;362: 211-2.
72. Dargie HJ, Cleland JGF, Leckie BJ, et al. Relation of arrhythmias and electrolyte abnormalities to survival in patients with severe chronic heart failure. Circulation 1987;75:98-107.
73. De Groote P, Dagorn J, Soudan B,Lamblin N, et al. B- type natriuretic peptide and peak exercise oxygen consumption provide independent information for risk stratification in patients with stable congestive heart failure. J Am Coll Cardiol 2004; 43: 1584-9.
74. Takeishi Y. Biomarkers in heart failure. Int Heart J 2014; 55:474-81.
75. Karaye KM, Sani MU. Factors associated with poor prognosis among patients admitted with heart failure in a Nigerian tertiary medical center: a cross-sectional study. BMC Cardiovascular Disorders. 2008;8(1).
76. Juilliere Y. Risk stratification in chronic heart failure. Annales de Cardiologie et d'Angéiologie. 2005;54(4):172–8.
77. Stevenson LW, Couper G, Natterson B, et al. Target heart failure populations for newer therapies. Circulation 1995;92(suppl):II74- II81.

78. Juillière Y, Danchin N, Briançon S, et al. Dilated cardiomyopathy: long-term follow-up and predictors of survival. Int J Cardiol 1988;21: 269-77.
79. Abramson SV, Burke JF, Kelly JJ. Pulmonary hypertension predicts mortality and morbidity in patients with dilated cardiomyopathy. Ann Intern Med 1992; 116: 888-95.
80. JuillièreY, Barbier G, Feldman L, et al. Additional predictive value of both left and right ventricular ejection fractions on long-term survival in idiopathic dilated cardiomyopathy. Eur Heart J 1997;18: 276-80.
81. Di Salvo TG, Mathier M, Semigran MJ, et al. Preserved right ventricular ejection fraction predicts exercise capacity and survival in advanced heart failure. J Am Coll Cardiol 1995;25: 1143-53.
82. De Groote P, Millaire A, Foucher-Hossein C, et al. Right ventricular ejection fraction is an independent predictor of survival in patients with moderate heart failure. J Am Coll Cardiol 1998;32: 948-54.
83. Alakoua N: Utilisation des amines vasopressives dans le service de cardiologie du CHU Yalgado Ouedraogo. Joseph Ki Zerbo University. 2014.

APPENDICES

<u>**FICHE DE COLLECTE - CAS**</u>

Fiche n°...........

Identité du patient décédé

Dossier clinique n°......... Date du décès: /_____/_____/________/

Age :.......... Sexe : F /___/ M/___/. Profession :...........

Niveau de vie : élevé /__/, Moyen /__/ Faible/__/

Antécédent d'insuffisance cardiaque : Oui /__/ durée (en mois) : /____/, Non /__/.

Durée d'hospitalisation (en jours) :........... jours

Données cliniques

Les facteurs de risque cardiovasculaires : Oui/__/ : Age (en années) /___/ HTA/__/ Diabète/__/ Tabac /___/ Dyslipidémie /__/ Obésité/__/ Alcool /__/ Autres :...........Non /__/

Comorbidités : Oui/__/. Insuffisance rénale /__/, Pneumopathies /___/, Anémie /___/ Autres :............... Non /__/

Stade de dyspnée selon la NYHA : stade I /__/ stade II /__/, stade III /__/, stade IV /__/

Toux : Oui /__/, Non /__/, Palpitations : Oui/__/, Non /__/. Douleur thoracique : Oui /__/.

Non /___/ Autres ....

La pression artérielle : PAS (en mm Hg) : /______/. PAD (en mm Hg) /____/

La fréquence cardiaque: /____/ BPM

Galop : Oui /__ / : Gauche /__/, Droit /__/, Gauche et Droit /__/. Non /__/

Signes d'ICD : Oui/__/ Non/__/

Etiologie de l'IC : HTA /__/, Ischémique /__/, valvulaire /__/, Toxique /__/, CMPP /__/

Autres :..

Données paracliniques

1- Biologie :

Groupe sanguin rhésus : A /__/, B /__/, O /__/, AB /__/.

Glycémie (en mmol/L) : /____/

Créatinine (en mmol/l) /_____/ DFG (ml/mn) /_____/

Urée (en mmol/l) /_____/

Taux d'Hémoglobine (en g/dl) /______/

Natrémie (en mmol/L) /_____/

Kaliémie (en mmol/l) /_____/

2- Electrocardiogramme

Fréquence cardiaque : /____/ CPM

TDR : Oui /__/. Non /__/

TDC : Oui /__/. Non /__/

3-Echocardiographie Doppler

a- Fonction ventriculaire gauche

DTDVG (en mm) : /_____/,

DTSVG (en mm) : /_____/

VTSVG : (en ml/m2) /_____/,

VTDVG (en ml/ m2) /_____/,

SIV (en mm) : /_____/,

PP (en mm) : /_____/,

FR (en %) : /_____/,

FE (en %) : /______/,

Trouble de la cinétique segmentaire : Oui: /__/. Non /__/.

Hypokinésie globale : Oui /___/. Non /___/

Thrombus intra cavitaire : Oui /__/ Non /__/.

Contraste spontané intra cavitaire : Oui /__/, Non /__/

Diamètre OG (en mm) : /_____/,

Surface OG (en mm2) : /______/,

IM : Oui /__/: grade I /__/, grade II /__/, grade III /__/, grade IV /__/. Non /__/

Pressions de remplissage VG : E/A : /____/

b- Fonction VD

Diamètre VD (en mm) : /_____/

TAPSE (en mm) : /____/,

Surface OD (en mm2) : /_____/,

VCI dilatée : Oui /__/ Non /__/

PAPS (en mmH) : /_____ /.

3- Traitement en hospitalisation :

a- Médicamenteux :

Diurétiques de l'anse : Oui /__/. Non /___/

Anti-aldostérone : Oui/__/. Non /___/

Béta bloquants Oui /__/. Non /___/

IEC : Oui /__/. Non /___/

ARAII : Oui /__/. Non /___/

Vasodilatateurs Oui /__/. Non /___/

Antiagrégant plaquettaire Oui /__/. Non /___/

anti-VitK : Oui /__/. Non /___/

Tonicardiaques Oui /__/. Non /___/

Statine : Oui/__/. Non /___/

Amiodarone Oui/__/. Non /___/

Trimetazidine Oui/__/. Non /___/

Autres...

Non médicamenteux

Choc électrique externe : Oui /__/, Non /__/

Pace Maker : Oui /__/, Non /__/

Causes probables de décés

TDR: Oui /__ / Non/__/,

TDC : Oui /__/ Non /__/

Choc cardiogénique : Oui /__/, Non /__/.

Autres :............................

Non précisé : /__/

FICHE DE COLLECTE - TEMOIN

Fiche n°...........

Identité du patient sortie vivant

Dossier clinique n°.......... Date d'hospitalisation : /____/_____/_________/

Age :........... Sexe : F /___/ M/___/. Profession :...........

Niveau de vie : élevé /__/, Moyen /__/ Faible/__/

Antécédent d'insuffisance cardiaque : Oui /__/ durée (en mois) : /____/,Non /__/.

Durée d'hospitalisation (en jours) :........... jours.

Données cliniques

Les facteurs de risque cardiovasculaires : Oui /__/ : Age (en années) /___/ HTA /__/

Diabète /__/ Tabac /___/ Dyslipidémie /__/ Obésité/ __/ Alcool /__/ Autres :.............Non/__/

Comorbidités : Oui/__/. Insuffisance rénale/__/, Pneumopathies /___/, Anémie /___/ Autres :............... Non /__/

Stade de dyspnée selon la NYHA : stade I /__/ stade II/__/, stade III /__/, stade IV /__/

Toux : Oui /__/, Non/__/, Palpitations : Oui/__/, Non /__/. Douleur thoracique : Oui /__/. Non/___/ Autres ....

La pression artérielle : PAS (en mm Hg) : /______/. PAD (en mmHg) /____/

La fréquence cardiaque: /____/ BPM

Galop : Oui /__ / : Gauche /__/, Droit /__/, Gauche et Droit /__/. Non /__/

Signes d'ICD : Oui /__/ Non /__/

Etiologie de l'IC : HTA /__/, Ischémique /__/, valvulaire /__/, Toxique /__/, CMPP /__/

Autres :...

Données paracliniques

1- Biologie :

Groupe sanguin rhésus : A /__/, B /__/, O /__/, AB /__/

Glycémie (en mmol/L) : /________/

Créatinine (en mmol/l) /________/ DFG (ml/mn) /_____/

Urée (en mmol/l) /_______/

Taux d'Hémoglobine (en g/dl) /_______/

Natrémie (en mmol/L) /_______/

Kaliémie (en mmol/l) /_______/

2- Electrocardiogramme

Fréquence cardiaque : /_____/ CPM

TDR : Oui /__/. Non /__/

TDC : Oui /__/. Non /__/

3- Echocardiographie Doppler

a- Fonction ventriculaire gauche

DTDVG (en mm) : /______/,

DTSVG (en mm) : /______/

VTSVG : (en ml/m2) /______/,

VTDVG (en ml/ m2) /______/,

SIV (en mm) : /______/,

PP (en mm) : /______/,

FR (en %) : /______/,

FE (en %) : /_______/,

Trouble de la cinétique segmentaire : Oui: /__/. Non /__/.

Hypokinésie globale : Oui /___/. Non /___/

Thrombus intra cavitaire : Oui /__/ Non /__/.

Contraste spontané intra cavitaire : Oui /__/, Non /__/

Diamètre OG (en mm) : /______/,

Surface OG (en mm2) : /_______/,

IM : Oui /__/: grade I /__/, grade II /__/, grade III /__/, grade IV /__/. Non /__/

Pressions de remplissage VG : E/A : /____/

b- Fonction ventriculaire droite

Diamètre VD (en mm) : /_______/

TAPSE (en mm) : /______/,

Surface OD (en mm2) : /_______/,

VCI dilatée : Oui /__/ Non /__/

PAPS (en mm Hg) : /_____ /,

4- Traitement en hospitalisation :

a- Médicamenteux :

Diurétiques de l'anse : Oui /__/. Non /___/

Anti-aldostérone : Oui /__/. Non /___/

Béta bloquants Oui /__/. Non /___/

IEC : Oui /__/. Non /___/

ARAII : Oui /__/. Non /___/

Vasodilatateurs Oui /__/. Non /___/

Antiagrégant plaquettaire Oui /__/. Non /___/

Anti-VitK : Oui /__/. Non /___/

Tonicardiaques Oui /__/. Non /___/

Statine : Oui /__/. Non /___/

Amiodarone Oui /__/. Non /___/

Trimetazidine Oui /__/. Non /___/

Autres..

b- Non médicamenteux

Choc électrique externe : Oui /__/, Non /__/

Pace Maker : Oui /__/, Non /__/

5- Traitement de sortie

Diurétiques de l'anse : Oui /__/. Non /___/

Anti-aldostérone : Oui /__/. Non /___/

Béta bloquants Oui /__/. Non /___/

IEC : Oui /__/. Non /___/

ARAII : Oui /__/. Non /___/

Vasodilatateurs Oui /__/. Non /___/

Antiagrégant plaquettaire Oui /__/. Non /___/

anti-VitK : Oui /__/. Non /___/

Tonicardiaques Oui /__/. Non /___/

Statine : Oui /__/. Non /___/

Amiodarone Oui /__/. Non /___/

Trimetazidine Oui /__/. Non /___/

Autres...

SUMMARY *:*

<u>Title</u>: Prognostic stratification in heart failure with reduced ejection fraction in black African subjects

Introduction: Heart failure is a serious disease with a high mortality rate. The aim of this study was to identify prognostic factors during heart failure. ***Method***: this was a case-control study conducted over a 24-month period (January 2017 to December 2018). Cases were patients hospitalized for heart failure with reduced ejection fraction who died during hospitalization, and controls were patients hospitalized for heart failure with reduced ejection fraction who were discharged alive. ***Results***: A personal history of heart failure was more common in cases (72%) than in controls (59%) (p< 0.001 and OR= 3.78). The mean length of hospital stay in our study population was 10.2 ± 0.5 days. Almost all cases (92.59%) were admitted with NYHA stage III and IV dyspnea (p= 0.004, OR= 2.8). Overall mean systolic blood pressure was 106.6 **±** 2.1 mmHg (80 mmHg ± 4.4 in cases and 115.4 mmHg ± 1.8 in controls, p=0.000 OR= 4.6). Overall mean glomerular filtration rate was 70.8 ± 2.7 ml/min (56± 4.7 ml/min in cases and 78.2 ± 3 ml/min in controls, p=0.001 OR= 4.6). Mean natraemia was 134.5 ± 0.6 mmol/L (129 ± 1 mmol/L in cases and 137 ± 0.5 mmol/L in controls). Hyponatremia was strongly associated with mortality (p=0.000, OR=5.5). Mean TAPSE was 15.1 ± 0.3 mm (13.9 ± 0.6 mm in cases and 15.7 ± 0.3 mm in controls, p= 0.02; 2.28).***Conclusion***: this study enabled us to identify factors associated with mortality in systolic heart failure. We have proposed a predictive score for this mortality.

Key words: mortality, heart failure, prognosis,

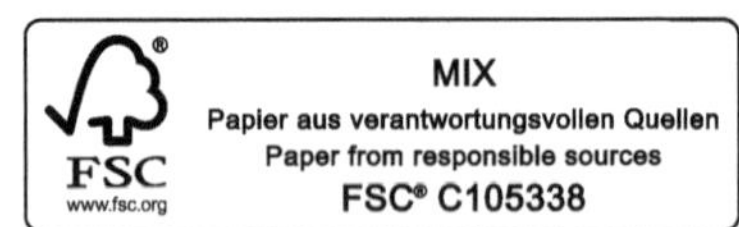

Printed by Books on Demand GmbH, Norderstedt / Germany